LONGITUDINAL RESEARCH IN THE
SOCIAL AND BEHAVIORAL SCIENCES
An Interdisciplinary Series

Series Editors:
Howard B. Kaplan, *Texas A&M University, College Station, Texas*
Adele Eskeles Gottfried, *California State University, Northridge, California*
Allen W. Gottfried, *California State University, Fullerton, California*

For further volumes:
http://www.springer.com/series/6236

Rolf Loeber · David P. Farrington

Young Homicide Offenders and Victims

Risk Factors, Prediction, and
Prevention from Childhood

With Contributions by:
Robert B. Cotter, Erin Dalton, Beth E. Ebel,
Darrick Jolliffe, Frederick P. Rivara,
Rebecca Stallings, and Magda Stouthamer-Loeber

Forewords by Kathleen M. Heide and Irvin Waller

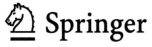 Springer

Rolf Loeber
Department of Psychiatry
University of Pittsburgh
Pittsburgh, PA 15213
USA
and
Free University
Amsterdam
The Netherlands
loeberr@upmc.edu

David P. Farrington
Cambridge University
Institute of Criminology
Cambridge CB3 9DA
UK
dpf1@cam.ac.uk

ISBN 978-1-4419-9948-1   e-ISBN 978-1-4419-9949-8
DOI 10.1007/978-1-4419-9949-8
Springer New York Dordrecht Heidelberg London

Library of Congress Control Number: 2011931973

Printed on acid-free paper

Springer is part of Springer Science+Business Media (www.springer.com)

Foreword by Kathleen M. Heide

In 1993, US attorney Janet Reno was asked at a news conference what was the greatest single crime problem facing the USA. Without a moment's hesitation, Ms. Reno said "youth violence" (Kantrowitz, 1993). For 10 consecutive years, arrests of young Americans, particularly juveniles, for violent crime, including homicide, had risen (Federal Bureau of Investigation, 1985–1994). Calculation of the absolute and relative levels of youth involvement in arrests for murder over the period 1958–1993 underscored the seriousness of the problem. The arrest rates for 15–19 year olds recorded in 1992 and 1993 were the highest for any age group during the 36-year-period under review (Smith & Feiler, 1995). Experts, including James A. Fox, Charles Patrick Ewing, and Al Blumstein predicted that youth involvement in homicide would continue to rise as the new millennium approached because the population of youths in the USA was on the increase (Heide, 1999).

Shortly after making that pronouncement, Janet Reno was a featured speaker at the American Society of Criminology conference. The large ballroom was filled to capacity. Ms. Reno thanked the audience of over 1,000 attendees for the important work that criminologists were doing. She emphasized that government needed our research to drive policy. However, she emphasized that government did not have the time to wait for long-drawn out research studies. The nation in times of crisis, such as the current one involving youth violence, needed answers fast.

The reality, as scholars know, is that good research based on adherence to strong scientific principles takes time. The present work by Rolf Loeber and David Farrington and their research team has been ongoing for over two decades. It is indeed extraordinary research and has the potential to pay huge dividends in terms of saving lives, decreasing human suffering, and improving the quality of life for many Americans.

Young Homicide Offenders and Victims: Risk Factors, Prediction, and Prevention from Childhood focuses on 37 convicted homicide offenders, 33 arrested homicide offenders who were not convicted, and 39 homicide victims. This scientific study by Loeber, Farrington, and their colleagues is groundbreaking in many respects: (1) longitudinal nature of the study; (2) large sample of subjects (1,517 males); (3) comparative analyses of convicted homicide offenders with homicide arrestees who were not convicted; (4) systematic study of both homicide offenders and victims; (5) utilization of several other control groups, including nonviolent boys, violent boys, and shooting victims; (6) exploration of 21 explanatory and 19 behavioral risk factors; (7) inclusion of both self-reported delinquency and official reports (arrests and convictions) for many different types of criminal behavior committed by boys up to age 14; (8) use of multiple informants (the youths, their parents, and teachers) and standardized measures when appropriate and available (e.g., California Achievement Test, Hollingshead Index based on parental education and occupational prestige, 1990 census data re: evaluation of neighborhoods, and Revised Diagnostic Interview Schedule for Children); (9) at least yearly assessments over a decade or more of dozens of background and behavioral development variables under investigation; and (10) application of an increasingly sophisticated series of analyses that included both bivariate and multivariate analyses. Each of these methodological design issues is noteworthy. To have all of them in one study is unparalleled and deserving of the highest accolades.

This book is one of many significant works to emerge from the Pittsburgh Youth Study (PYS), a prospective longitudinal study that consisted of repeated assessments of three community cohorts of inner city boys. The study began in 1987 when the boys were in the first, fourth, and seventh grades in Pittsburgh public schools. Participation by the boys and their parents in the PYS was exceedingly high, ranging from 84 to 86% across the three cohorts. In an effort to increase the number of high-risk males in the follow-up cohort, the researchers devised a screening instrument using information from the boys, their parents, and teachers to identify the 30% of the boys that were most antisocial. Another 30% of the boys were randomly selected from the remaining 70%. The extensiveness of the follow-up available varied by cohort. The youngest cohort ($n=503$) was assessed 18 times from ages 7 through 19, and the oldest cohort ($n=506$), 16 times, from ages 13 to 25. The middle cohort ($n=508$) was assessed only seven times, from ages 10 to 13. There were no gaps in the assessment intervals. Accordingly, as noted by the authors in Chap. 2, "the study is uniquely poised to investigate individuals' onset of delinquency and substance abuse, and individual's continuation of and desistance from these behaviors."

Longitudinal studies exist that have investigated the difficulties and mental health issues faced by adolescents during their development. Some of these research efforts have examined youth involvement in substance abuse, delinquency, and high-risk behavior (e.g., Brunswick, n.d.; Resnick et al., 1997). The present longitudinal study stands alone in having the follow-up data to assess, from its initial cohort, a sample of boys who were subsequently arrested and convicted of murder.

Among those convicted, offenders ranged in age from 15 through 26 years at the time of the killing. Approximately 72% were in their teenage years when the murder occurred (19% were under age 18). All but two of the convicted murderers (94%) were under age 25 at the time of the homicidal event. Recent research has indicated that the part of the brain most associated with critical thinking and decision making (prefrontal cortex) does not complete its development until the early 20s, and, perhaps, not until about age 25 (Beckman, 2004; Giedd, 2004).

Accordingly, the findings of this study may be appropriately discussed with reference to the available literature on juvenile, adolescent, and youth homicide.

Although there is an extensive body of research available on youth homicide, the literature has suffered from several serious limitations that the present work has overcome. The literature on juvenile and adolescent murderers has consisted predominantly of studies with small samples. Research studies of homicide by juveniles and other young offenders have been primarily clinical in focus (Heide, 2003). Samples have often been convenience samples, such as youths referred to mental health professionals for evaluation (e.g., Bender, 1959; Bailey, 1996; Corder, Ball, Haizlip, Rollins, & Beaumont, 1976; Cornell, Benedek, & Benedek, 1989; Myers, Scott, Burgess, & Burgess, 1995), those referred to juvenile or adult court (Roe-Sepowitz, 2009; Sorrells, 1977; Zagar, Busch, Grove, & Hughes, 2009), inmates incarcerated for murder or attempted murder that they committed as juveniles (e.g., Heide, Spencer, Thompson, & Solomon, 2001; Hill-Smith, Hugo, Hughes, Fonagy, & Hartman, 2002) or juvenile murderers on death row (Lewis et al., 1988).

Given their largely retrospective nature, these earlier works can rarely speak authoritatively about causal factors. With the exception of a few studies, such as those recently published by Zagar and his colleagues (Zagar et al., 2009), prior studies have not used control groups so it is unknown whether factors identified as defining young homicide offenders would apply to other groups, such as violent offenders or delinquent youth in general.

Previous studies of young murderers, however, have made important contributions in suggesting factors that appear to be associated with killings committed by young people. These include psychological disorders, particularly mood disorders (depression), behavioral disorders (Attention Deficit Hyperactivity Disorder, Oppositional Defiant Disorder, Conduct Disorder), anxiety disorders (Post-traumatic Stress Disorder), and substance abuse and/or dependence. In addition to mental health problems, family problems, including parental substance abuse and criminality, domestic violence, child maltreatment, and broken homes, have frequently been found in the backgrounds of young homicide offenders. Truancy, low school achievement, dropping out, expulsion from school, and a history of antisocial and criminal behavior have been identified among youths involved in murder. The extent to which generalizations can be drawn from these studies to the population of youth homicide offenders has been unknown. With the publication of *Young Homicide Offenders and Victims: Risk Factors, Prediction, and Prevention from Childhood*, many of the questions about which variables distinguish young convicted killers from other groups of their peers, such as unconvicted homicide arrestees, violent offenders, and homicide victims, can now be answered.

Several analyses of juvenile homicide offenders have been undertaken by teams of researchers using the Supplementary Homicide Report database (Heide, Solomon, Sellers, & Chan, 2011). Information on murders (criminal homicide and nonnegligent manslaughter) and homicide arrestees is voluntarily submitted to the FBI's Uniform Crime Reports Program by law enforcement agencies on murders known to them. However, this database, although national in scope, is limited to basic victim and offender demographic information (age, race, gender, victim–offender relationship), case-related variables (weapon used, codefendants, situation type, homicide circumstance), and incident-related information (state, urban level, population density, offense year, etc.). These studies are valuable in describing the correlates of youth homicide. The data set, however, does not contain variables that measure social or behavioral characteristics of victims and offenders. Given the cross-sectional nature of these analyses, conclusions about causal factors involved in youth homicide are not possible.

The present work, unlike earlier ones, can speak confidently to causation. Given the assessments of youth taken initially at 6 month and then yearly intervals, the temporal order of events could be measured. The PYS data set stands alone in providing causal information about the early risk factors and problem behaviors of boys who later became homicide offenders or victims. Early risk factors included, for example, factors involving the youth's birth, school performance, psychopathic traits, mood indicators, measures related to family functioning, child-rearing practices, SES, and bad neighborhood. Behavioral risk factors included indicators of conduct disorder, attitudes favorable to delinquency and substance abuse, measures of difficulties with a parent, involvement with delinquent or substance abusing peers, attitudinal and behavioral measures of school difficulties, and measures relating to weapons, gang involvement, and drug use and selling. Most of these data came from parents and the boys. Information was also obtained from the boys' teachers and educational achievement tests.

Predictors of homicide offending were not limited to explanatory and behavioral risk factors. In an effort to improve on the accuracy of the prediction of convicted homicide offenders, self-reported offending and official reports of delinquent acts committed up to age 14 obtained from police and the courts were measured. Criminal risk factors assessed included self-reported crimes involving violence, property, drug use and selling, and other deviance, such as using alcohol or tobacco, or being drunk in public. Arrests and convictions for violence, property crimes, or other crimes, such as drugs, mischief/disorder, other/conspiracy, or any other arrest prior to age 15 were also included.

The analyses undertaken by the authors were colossal in nature, meticulous in execution, and unprecedented in many respects. Their innovative approach to studying homicides by young offenders uncovered many important findings with potentially significant implications for theory, policy, and future research. The authors' decision to divide homicide arrestees into two groups (those who were convicted and those who were not convicted), for example, resulted in several interesting findings. Surprisingly, analyses revealed little overlap between the two groups. The groups tended to differ from one another with respect to explanatory and behavioral risk factors. Socioeconomic factors (broken family, family on welfare, young mother, unemployed mother, low socioeconomic status) were more characteristic of convicted homicide offenders. In contrast, behavioral factors (truancy, low school achievement, low school motivation, nonphysical aggression) were more associated with homicide arrestees.

One of the most fascinating findings to emerge from making the distinction between homicide arrestees and convicted homicide offenders involved race.

Race was not significantly related to convicted homicide offenders after the effects of other risk variables were controlled. However, when homicide arrestees were combined with convicted homicide offenders, African American race remained a significant predictor of combined homicide offenders. This research calls into question the practice frequently employed by researchers of using homicide arrestees as accurate measures of homicide offenders. In this case, combining 33 homicide arrestees with 37 convicted homicide offenders increased the sample size in these analyses from 37 to 70. The present research suggests that at least among urban African American adolescents and young adults, the percentage of homicide arrestees who will be found guilty of homicide may be significantly less than the number arrested, perhaps, by as much as by 40% or more. The authors offered several reasons for the large number of homicide arrestees not being convicted. These included lack of evidence, racial discrimination, or witness intimidation by homicide arrestees. Clearly more research is needed.

This study found that similar proportions of the PYS sample became convicted homicide offenders (2.4%) and homicide victims (2.6%). Interestingly, the convicted homicide offenders more closely resembled the homicide victims than the arrested homicide offenders. As noted by the authors, the strongest predictors of homicide victims tended to be the same as the strongest predictors of convicted homicide offenders. Both groups had committed serious delinquency prior to age 15. However, unlike convicted homicide offenders, race continued to predict homicide victims after controlling for the effects of all explanatory risk factors. The authors noted that this result is likely due to the fact that 37 of the 39 victims were African American.

One of the most intriguing analyses undertaken by the authors involved determining whether a dose–response relationship existed between the number of explanatory, behavioral, and criminal risk factors and the probability of becoming a convicted homicide offender. The researchers found that the integrated homicide risk score for the prediction of convicted homicide offenders from the whole population indicated that the probability of becoming a homicide offender increased as the number of risk factors increased. However, the false-positive error rate (Type 1 error) was very high, indicating that many individuals identified as potential homicide offenders did not commit homicide. At the same time, the false-negative error rate (Type 2) was moderately high, suggesting that, perhaps, as many as 40% of homicide offenders were missed.

Similar analyses showed that the probability of becoming a homicide victim also increased as the number of risk factors increased. The risk factors predicted homicide victims almost as well as convicted homicide offenders. However, once again, issues of Type 1 and 2 errors were present.

Although replication in research is both desirable and necessary, findings in this study appear generalizable to the population of young urban males arrested and convicted of homicide in the USA. As Loeber and Farrington demonstrated, findings related to the homicide offenders and their victims did not appear to be restricted to the Pittsburgh area. The murder offenders and victims in the PYS resembled their counterparts in the Allegheny County in which Pittsburgh is located in terms of gender, race, weapon use, neighborhood disadvantage, homicide motive, and criminal record. Comparisons between PYS homicide offenders and their victims with their urban counterparts in the USA, although limited, suggested many similarities between the groups. One of the most disturbing similarities found on the county, city, and national levels involved the exceedingly high overrepresentation of African American young males among both homicide offenders and victims.

The authors tackled the controversial issues raised by their findings. They addressed the high proportion of PYS youths who engaged in violent behavior and analyzed predictors of violent offenders who did not become homicide offenders or victims, or shooting victims. They noted the high involvement of African American males as both homicide offenders and victims, and offered explanations for their disparate findings regarding the significance of race. Loeber and Farrington discussed the theoretical aspects of the development of violence and homicide offending, with special attention given to the "Integrated Cognitive Antisocial Potential" (ICAP) theory designed to explain offending by lower class males (Farrington, 2003).

The authors proposed the use of screening instruments to identify youths at high risk of killing or being killed. They argued that these instruments should assess needs in addition to risks. The emphasis, they maintained, must be on helping children and their families, and not on stigmatizing and punishing them.

The findings reported in *Young Homicide Offenders and Victims: Risk Factors, Prediction, and Prevention from Childhood* make a compelling argument for intervention. One finding that may surprise many readers is that the homicide offenders in the PYS had received a variety of services for their mental and behavioral problems. Obviously these interventions were not successful in preventing the boys from subsequently committing homicide. Loeber and Farrington argued persuasively that implementing interventions based on programs that have proven success records and are targeted at high-risk populations on a national level is needed. Using simulated models, the authors showed that these programs could save many lives and could result in saving billions of dollars due to reduced incarceration costs.

The reduction in human suffering by families, friends, and other survivors of both homicide victims and homicide offenders that would flow from the savings of lives is incalculable. The elimination of terror that holds countless men, women, and children, particularly those who live in poor communities, hostage in their own homes is not just a lofty goal. *Young Homicide Offenders and Victims: Risk Factors, Prediction, and Prevention from Childhood* provides a blueprint for the USA to achieve a healthier and safer society for all its members.

Kathleen M. Heide
Professor of Criminology
College of Behavioral and Community Sciences
University of South Florida

References

Bailey, S. (1996). Adolescents who murder. *Journal of Adolescence, 19*, 19–39.
Beckman, M. (2004). Crime, culpability, and the adolescent brain. *Science, 305*, 596–599.
Bender, L. (1959). Children and adolescents who have killed. *American Journal of Psychiatry, 116*, 510–513.
Brunswick, A. F. (n.d.) *Harlem longitudinal study of urban black youth, 1968–1994.* Retrieved: http://hdl.handle.net/1902.1/00845 UNF:4:6,128:zmyHvveCO6LrHnfxycgV4w+PR/2Hc4b9 hT4r1GnOoBo= Murray Research Archive [Distributor] V2 [Version].
Corder, B. F., Ball, B. C., Haizlip, T. M., Rollins, R., & Beaumont, R. (1976). Adolescent parricide: A comparison with other adolescent murder. *American Journal of Psychiatry, 133*(8), 957–961.
Cornell, D. G., Benedek, E. P., & Benedek, D. M. (1989). A typology of juvenile homicide offenders. In E. P. Benedek & D. G. Cornell (Eds.), *Juvenile homicide* (pp. 59–84). Washington, DC: American Psychiatric Press.
Federal Bureau of Investigation. (1985–1994*). Crime in the United States (1984–1993).* Washington, DC: U.S. Government Printing Office.
Giedd, J. N. (2004). Structural magnetic resonance imaging of the adolescent brain. *Annals of the New York Academy of Sciences, 1021*, 105–109.
Heide, K. M., Solomon, E. P., Sellers, B. G., & Chan. H. C. (2011). Male and female juvenile homicide offenders: An empirical analysis of U.S. arrests by offender age. *Feminist Criminology, 6*(1), 3–31.
Heide, K. M., Spencer, E., Thompson, A., & Solomon, E. P. (2001). Who's in, who's out, and who's back: Follow-up data on 59 juveniles incarcerated for murder or attempted murder in the early 1980s. *Behavioral Sciences and the Law, 19*, 97–108.
Hill-Smith, A. J., Hugo, P., Hughes, P., Fonagy, P., & Hartman, D. (2002). Adolescent murderers: Abuse and adversity in childhood. *Journal of Adolescence, 25*, 221–230.
Kantrowitz, B. (1993, Aug 2). Teen violence – Wild in the streets. *Newsweek*, pp. 40–46.
Lewis, D. O., Pincus, J. H., Bard, B., Richardson, E., Feldman, M., Prichep, L. S., et al. (1988). Neuropsychiatric, psychoeducational, and family characteristics of 14 juveniles condemned to death in the United States. *American Journal of Psychiatry, 145*, 584–589.
Myers, W. C., Scott, K., Burgess, A. W., & Burgess, A. G. (1995). Psychopathology, biopsychosocial factors, crime characteristics, and classification of 25 homicidal youths. *Journal of the American Academy of Child and Adolescent Psychiatry, 34*, 1483–1489.
Resnick, M. D., Bearman, P. S., Blum, R. W., Bauman, K. F., Harris, K. M., Jones, J., et al. (1997). Protecting adolescents from harm: Findings from the National Longitudinal Study on Adolescent Health. *JAMA, 278*(10), 823–832.
Roe-Sepowitz, D. E. (2009).Comparing male and female juveniles charged with homicide: Child maltreatment, substance abuse and crime details. *The Journal of Interpersonal Violence, 24*(4), 601–617.
Smith, M. D. & Feiler, S. M. (1995). Absolute and relative involvement in homicide offending: Contemporary youth and the baby boom cohorts. *Violence and Victims, 10*, 327–333.
Sorrells, J. M., Jr. (1977). Kids who kill. *Crime & Delinquency, 16*, 152–161.
Zagar, R. J., Busch, K. G., Grove, W. M., & Hughes, J. R. (2009). Summary of studies of abused infants and children later homicidal, and homicidal, assaulting later homicidal, and sexual homicidal youth and adults. *Psychological Reports, 104*, 17–45.

Foreword by Irvin Waller

This book faces the stark reality that rates of homicide in the USA far exceed those of any other rich democratic nation. Drs Loeber and Farrington are internationally the undisputed gurus of scientific analysis of how young boys develop into serious adult offenders and of what might cause those levels of violence. In this book, they have done it again by carefully and rigorously showing which negative life experiences predispose young males to becoming killers or the killed – the ultimate crimes.

Starting with some key statistics, they show how certain young African American males grow up to kill or be killed. They point to the importance of being born to young mothers, experiencing family break-up and suffering a family on welfare. They recall how drug dealing, hand guns, and school failure are just some of the experiences that differentiate those who kill or get killed from those in the same neighborhoods who survive. These are familiar territory to those who have worked to stop crime, but they take on a special importance when focused on homicide.

But the book does not stop there, since they have chapters that focus on the potential return on investment from tackling some of the negative life experiences at very early stages. One of their chapters convincingly shows how Nationwide implementation for at-risk families of the Nurse Home Visitation Program and the Perry Pre-school Program will each prevent between 20 and 24% of all homicides, reducing the cost of incarceration by about $3–6 billion per year and an estimated $5–10 billion in the costs of loss of life.

At a time when voters are calling for cutting deficits and ensuring taxpayers' money is used responsibly, these models provide a basis for significant reallocations. Indeed, the Obama administration has already started with $8 billion over the next 10 years for nurse home visitation. But the evidence in this book justifies a more significant rebalancing of budgets from overspending on an incarceration industry whose growth has exceeded that of many governmental sectors. Currently, the US incarcerates one in four of all prisoners worldwide and still has the highest rates of homicide. Reallocating 10% of the $70 billion each year spent on incarceration would rapidly bring the US annual rates of homicide closer to those of other rich democratic nations. That is saving 3,000 or likely many more lives each year. The evidence to justify these investments is in this book.

In the last chapter, the gurus open the debate on ways to get more investment in programs that are effective in reducing violence. They discuss some important next steps, including the implementation in Pittsburgh of Stop Now and Plan (SNAP). Earlier evaluations of this program show considerable promise and so likely would result also in reductions in violence and homicides nationwide.

But much more is possible, if the conclusions can be framed appropriately for legislators at all government levels. Indeed, this book becomes available at an opportune time. The World Health Organization is planning to follow-up its seminal report on preventing violence with a report that will update the evidence and assess the extent to which countries are implementing strategies that prevent violence.

There are a growing number of governments who are investing in evidence strategies that include a government responsibility center to use evidence such as that in this book. This interest comes from books such as *Less Law, More Order: The Truth about Reducing Crime* that take the conclusions from the work of the gurus, frame it for government in terms of reducing numbers of crime victims, argue the case for the return on investment, and establish permanent strategies and responsibility centers to shift funds from what does not work to what does.

This book is an important addition to the scientific literature that provides a further evidence base for shifting policies from eighteenth-century thinking about punishment to twenty-first century action to stop homicides and violence. If you start with the conclusions from the gurus, you will be drawn back quickly to read the chapters that form the basis for what is a very hopeful and overdue vision that homicide is eminently preventable if you use the Loeber and Farrington science to make policy. This is not just for academic journals but the real world of stopping crime and protecting victims.

Irvin Waller
President, International Organization for Victim Assistance
Founding and Past Executive Director, International Centre
for Prevention of Crime, affiliated with the United Nations
Professor of Criminology, University of Ottawa

Preface

Among the books published on homicide, this volume is the first to use prospective longitudinal data to predict homicide offenders and victims from childhood risk factors and to consider preventive interventions for homicide in a systematic manner. Each book has its own history and this volume has a long history. When faced with increasing numbers of homicide offenders and homicide victims in the Pittsburgh Youth Study, the second author convinced the first author of the need to undertake extensive analyses and write this volume. Many interfering tasks occurred over the years and the volume only gradually took shape with long intermissions.

Work on this book was supported by grants 96-MU-FX-0012 and 2005-JK-FX-0001 from the Office of Juvenile Justice and Delinquency Prevention (OJJDP), grants MH 50778 and 73941 from the National Institute of Mental Health, grant No. 11018 from the National Institute on Drug Abuse, a grant from the Department of Health of the Commonwealth of Pennsylvania, and a grant from the Centers for Disease Control (administered through OJJDP). Analyses in Chap. 8 were supported by a Robert Wood Johnson Foundation Grant to Dr. Frederick P. Rivara. However, this sponsor has not participated in the design and conduct of the study, collection, management, analysis, interpretation of the data, preparation, review, of approval of the report. Dr. Beth Ebel has had full access to all of the data and takes responsibility for the integrity of the data and the accuracy of the analysis in Chap. 8.

Points of view or opinions in this book are those of the authors and do not necessarily represent the official position or policies of any of the aforementioned agencies. We are particularly grateful to Maureen Brown and Jennifer Wilson for their efficient administrative help, and to Rebecca Stallings for her most efficient preparation of the data and checking of the constructs. We also thank the following individuals for their most generous help and advice: Mark Berg, Alfred Blumstein, Matt Durose, Anthony Fabio, Megan Good, James C. Howell, Patrick A. Langan, Janet L. Lauritsen, Dustin A. Pardini, James Rieland, Richard B. Rosenfeld, Howard N. Snyder, Brandon C. Welsh, Helene R. White, Norman White, and James Williams. Foremost, we are very grateful to the staff and the participants of the Pittsburgh Youth Study who laid the foundation for this volume. In addition, we owe much to our co-authors: Robert B. Cotter, Erin Dalton,

Beth E. Ebel, Darrick Jolliffe, Dustin A. Pardini, Frederick P. Rivara, Rebecca Stallings, and Magda Stouthamer-Loeber. We are very much indebted to Magda Stouthamer-Loeber for supervising and guiding the study over decades and for her unwavering confidence that we would complete this book.

Pittsburgh, PA   Rolf Loeber
Cambridge, UK   David P. Farrington

Endorsements

This is a fascinating, pioneering book. Based on results from the Pittsburgh Youth Study, it identifies childhood risk factors that predict involvement in homicide as offenders and victims, and it offers provocative simulations of the potential impacts of possible prevention strategies. The authors' sophisticated analyses demonstrate convincingly the considerable value of prospective longitudinal data for enhancing our understanding of the etiology and control of lethal violence.

Steven F. Messner, Ph.D.
Distinguished Teacher Professor, Department of Sociology,
University at Albany, SUNY
President, American Society of Criminology

How do homicide offenders differ from other violent offenders with respect to early-life and more proximate risk factors? How do homicide offenders differ from homicide victims? Is it possible to predict, years in advance, who will kill or be killed? Until now, homicide researchers could only speculate about the answers to these and related questions, or the answers were based on crude and often unreliable data. This book changes the game in violence research. Analyzing richly detailed data from a community sample of boys studied from early childhood into young adulthood, Loeber and Farrington dissect the developmental pathways that lead to lethal violence and propose interventions to ameliorate the early-life risk factors that otherwise lead predictably to violence and death. The analysis is masterful, the prose is readable, and the achievement is nothing short of stunning. This book is required reading for veteran researchers, students, criminal justice and public health professionals, and anyone who wants to know what cutting edge research on a critical public problem looks like.

Richard Rosenfeld, Ph.D.
Curators Professor of Criminology and Criminal Justice,
University of Missouri-St. Louis
Past President, American Society of Criminology

Beginning with Wolfgang's classic Patterns in Criminal Homicide, many important books on homicide have followed but none has recently emerged as a turning point in the field. That is, until now. Loeber and Farrington's volume is a collection of firsts in many respects, primarily because it is the first to use prospective longitudinal data to predict homicide offenders and victims from childhood risk factors as well as to consider prevention/intervention efforts in great detail. In very short order, Young Homicide Offenders and Victims: Development, Risk Factors, and Prediction from Childhood will become one of those key books that sits on the desks and shelves of students, academics, practitioners, and policy makers alike. But, unlike some others, this is one that will be read, reread, and learned from in many respects.

Alex R. Piquero, Ph.D.
Gordon P. Waldo Professor of Criminology
Florida State University

This book will stand the test of time as a landmark homicide study. Principally, it is the first of its kind to analyze the development of a representative sample of homicide offenders and victims over the life course, from childhood to adulthood. Moreover, the researchers are two of the most renowned developmental criminologists in the world.

James C. Howell, Ph.D.
Senior Research Associate
National Gang Center

Contents

1   **Young Male Homicide Offenders and Victims:**
     Current Knowledge, Beliefs, and Key Questions 1
     Rolf Loeber and David P. Farrington

2   **The Pittsburgh Youth Study** 19
     Rolf Loeber, David P. Farrington, and Rebecca Stallings

3   **Homicide Offenders and Victims in the USA, Pennsylvania,**
     Pittsburgh, and the Pittsburgh Youth Study 37
     Rolf Loeber, Erin Dalton, and David P. Farrington

4   **Early Risk Factors for Convicted Homicide**
     Offenders and Homicide Arrestees 57
     David P. Farrington and Rolf Loeber

5   **Prediction of Homicide Offenders Out of Violent Boys** 79
     David P. Farrington and Rolf Loeber

6   **Early Risk Factors for Homicide Victims and Shooting Victims** 95
     David P. Farrington and Rolf Loeber

7   **Homicide Offenders Speak** 115
     Darrick Jolliffe, Rolf Loeber, David P. Farrington,
     and Robert B. Cotter

8   **Modeling the Impact of Preventive Interventions**
     on the National Homicide Rate 123
     Beth E. Ebel, Frederick P. Rivara, Rolf Loeber,
     and Dustin A. Pardini

9   **Modeling the Impact of Interventions on Local Indicators**
       of Offending, Victimization, and Incarceration 137
       Rolf Loeber and Rebecca Stallings

10   **Conclusions and Implications** 153
       Rolf Loeber and David P. Farrington

References 187

Index 197

About the Authors

Rolf Loeber is Professor of Psychiatry, Psychology, and Epidemiology at the Western Psychiatric Institute and Clinic, School of Medicine, University of Pittsburgh, and Professor of Juvenile Delinquency and Social Development, Free University, Amsterdam, Netherlands. He is co-chair of the U.S. National Institute of Justice Study Group on Transitions from Juvenile Delinquency to Adult Crime and co-chair of the U.S. Centers for Disease Control Expert Panel on Protective Factors against Youth Violence. He is Co-director of the Life History Program and is principal investigator of three longitudinal studies, the Pittsburgh Youth Study, the Developmental Trends Study, and the Pittsburgh Girls Study. He has published widely in the fields of juvenile antisocial behavior and delinquency, substance use, and mental health problems (more than 215 peer-reviewed papers, 114 book chapters and other papers, and 9 books).

David P. Farrington, O.B.E., is Professor of Psychological Criminology at the Institute of Criminology, Cambridge University, and Adjunct Professor of Psychiatry at Western Psychiatric Institute and Clinic, University of Pittsburgh. He is co-chair of the U.S. National Institute of Justice Study Group on Transitions from Juvenile Delinquency to Adult Crime and co-chair of the U.S. Centers for Disease Control Expert Panel on Protective Factors against Youth Violence. His major research interest is in developmental criminology, and he is Director of the Cambridge Study in Delinquent Development, which is a prospective longitudinal survey of over 400 London males from age 8 to age 48. In addition to over 500 published journal articles and book chapters on criminological and psychological topics, he has published over 75 books, monographs and government publications.

Chapter 1
Young Male Homicide Offenders and Victims: Current Knowledge, Beliefs, and Key Questions

Rolf Loeber and David P. Farrington

This volume deals with three categories of individuals involved in murder: convicted homicide offenders, homicide arrestees, and violent boys. The volume also studies two categories of victims: homicide victims and shooting victims. Highly unusual for homicide studies, all five categories of individuals were studied from childhood onwards, thus years before they became a killer, were arrested for a killing, became violent, or were killed or wounded.

Most people are never or rarely directly confronted with killings, other than on television, video games, or in movies. However, for some segments of the population, killings are real and close by. In August 2008, the first author of this volume took a taxi ride with one of his favorite (African American) cab drivers, who told him how his family and friends had suffered from recent homicides in Pittsburgh. Here follows a summary of what the driver said:

Homicide – that is exactly what has happened to my family just recently. May I say this? When you see killings in a movie one can be 95% desensitized to the reality of the permanency of the act. When watching this evil act being reported in the news the desensitizing is lessened and the sensitivity becomes greater the closer the dastardly deed is done in relation to where one lives and also to whom one may know indirectly, whether it be the victim or the perp[etrator], the doer of said evil deed. But on July 4, 2008 there was a direct relationship with the reality of the permanency of a homicide – human killer of another. My brother-in law was shot and killed at approximately 4:00 in the morning while asleep and the woman that was with him was also shot and killed. This beloved father, husband, son, brother, uncle, and friend was permanently taken away from us by this evil act. A week later this permanent act surfaced again when my brother-in law's nephew from his wife's side was shot and killed while at work by a lost human killer trying to rob the restaurant. Homicides continue with close relations to my family. A few days after the previous killing a young man who had graduated from high school with my granddaughter, who she knew well, had been shot and killed possibly by another young man that everyone in my family knew. And now a few days later a friend of my oldest son was shot and killed by another lost individual simply because the victim would not give this perp[etrator] a ride. This young man, the victim, was finishing college while working. But yet Death in the form of homicide was not yet done although moving away from family connections. The string of human life destruction continued. Two 45-year-old men coming back to Pittsburgh to visit with their families, after recently moving away to West Virginia or just Virginia, they were shot and killed while driving in their truck in Homewood by some young thugs for no apparent reason. This has been a very darkened July for my wife and her brother and sisters and relatives and myself also for the many other families here in Pittsburgh and for the rest of our days will never be without a void and a pain of missing a loved one because of the selfish evilness of lost "Homicideans" [human killers] and the selfishness of the NRA [National Rifle Association].

This personal account shows the pervasiveness of killings in Pittsburgh and the number of people directly and indirectly affected by the murders. An informal survey of local young (mostly African American) people in Pittsburgh in 2010 reported that nearly 80% had family or friends wounded or killed by gun violence (Kalson, 2010).

Violence and homicide remain a persisting and serious problem in many parts of the world (Harrendorf, Heiskanen, & Malby, 2010; Krug, Dahlberg, Mercy, Zwi, & Lozano, 2002). In 2008, over 7,000 (7,305) young people between the ages of 15 and 29 were murdered in the USA, that is on average 20 each day of the year (Federal Bureau of Investigation, 2008). Efforts by the criminal justice system to reduce fatal and nonfatal violence have centered on policing policies, incarceration, control of the illegal drug trade, and legally restricting minors' and felons' access to firearms. These policies are said to have been partly responsible for the drop in homicide rates after the peak in the early 1990s (Blumstein, Rivara, & Rosenfeld, 2000). However, the policies have not reduced homicide rates by and of young people in the USA to a level that is comparable to those of most other developed countries (Farrington, Langan, & Tonry, 2004). To put the yearly toll of murdered young people in perspective, each year more than twice as many young people are killed as the number of deaths resulting from the attack on the World Trade Center in New York on September 11, 2001.

For the 15- to 24-year-old group, homicide is the second leading cause of death, after accidents and before suicide (Hoyert, Arias, Smith, Murphy, & Kochanek, 2001, Table 8). Homicide especially concerns African American young men, both as offenders and as victims (Anderson & Smith, 2002; Cook & Laub, 1998; Fox & Zawitz, 2007). Health and justice records show that both homicide victims and homicide offenders are rare under age 15, are quite prevalent at ages 15–29, and then decline from age 30 onwards.

This book is about several groups of vulnerable individuals. First, it deals with young male killers, who have been studied for many years before they murdered someone. We will also examine individuals who were arrested for homicide but not convicted. Second, this book deals with victims of homicide and aspects of their lives many years before they were killed. We will also look into the background of victims of shootings who survived. As detailed later, this type of prospective study of vulnerable individuals is much more informative than the typical homicide study that retrospectively attempts to piece together after-the-fact the possible circumstances over many years that might have led to a person committing murder (e.g., Goodman, Mercy, Layde, & Thacker, 1988; Miethe & Regoeczi, 2004; Wikström & Treiber, 2009).

Although some studies (e.g., Bailey, 1996) have used matching of murderers and controls (i.e., individuals who did not murder), these publications are methodologically weak because they depend on inconsistently collected information in archives and on imperfect recall of past events by offenders, their relatives, and friends. Also, comparisons between extreme groups (i.e., homicide offenders and nonoffenders) tend to produce artificially strong results (e.g., Zagar, Busch, Grove, & Hughes, 2009). As a consequence, case–control publications provide inadequate information about antecedents, predictors, and causes of homicide. Critically, they do not have adequate information about individuals who may have resembled homicide offenders at a young age, but who did not subsequently commit homicide.

These disadvantages do not apply to the Pittsburgh Youth Study (or PYS in short), which for the first time in the annals of homicide studies prospectively collected information from childhood into early adulthood about the lives and conditions under which young men grew up in a mid-sized city, some of whom became homicide offenders, some of whom became victims of homicide, and most of whom became neither. The PYS is a prospective longitudinal follow-up study of 1,517 Pittsburgh young males from childhood to adulthood (for details, see Chap. 2).

Why would Pittsburgh data be relevant for state or national issues concerning homicide offending and homicide victimization? In Chap. 3, it is shown that conditions associated with homicide offenses (such as the use of guns, involvement of gangs and drugs, male against male arguments, African American young males victimizing African American young males) for participants in the PYS at the local level of Pittsburgh are very similar for Allegheny County in which Pittsburgh is situated, the Commonwealth of Pennsylvania, and the USA.

Before presenting the results of our investigation in Chaps. 2–9, we briefly present background information about homicide offending by young men in the USA.

Homicide Offenders, Violent Offenders, and Their Victims

Compared to other developed countries, the USA has one of the highest rates of homicide in the Western World (Farrington et al., 2004; Roth, 2009) and this differential is highest for homicides among unrelated adults. In comparison, rates of intimate homicides in the USA are not materially different from many other countries (Roth, 2009). In recent memory, the USA experienced a peak in violence and homicide offending. The rates of homicide offenders and victims in ages 13–17 and 18–24 increased from 1985 to a peak in 1993 and then declined (Cook & Laub, 1998, p. 45; Fox & Zawitz, 2007). For ages 18–24, the rates at the peak in 1993 were almost double the rates in 1985; for ages 13–17, the rates at the peak in 1993 were almost triple the rates in 1985. Much of the increase in violence reflected the deaths of African American youth rather than Caucasian or other youth (Harms & Snyder, 2004; Berg, 2010. Personal communication based on the supplemental homicide reports, 1976–2005). For ages 18–24, the peak homicide offending rate in 1993 was 280 per 100,000 for African Americans and 30 per 100,000 for Caucasians; the peak homicide victimization rate in 1993 was 190 per 100,000 for African Americans and 20 per 100,000 for Caucasians (Cook & Laub, 1998, p. 47).

In Chap. 3, we show that the rates of homicide offending and victimization in the PYS are higher than the peak national rate in 1993, and even higher when the rate over the life-time (in this case, over the first three decades of life) is considered. Thus, the problem of homicide has not gone down in a city such as Pittsburgh. In fact, as shown in Chap. 3, the problem has gradually become worse over the past decades.

Not all generations of youth, whether African American or Caucasian (the two major ethnic groups in the City of Pittsburgh), are equally at risk of homicide offending or homicide victimization. The differential between the two racial groups has dramatically increased after 1985, peaking in 1993, and although lower subsequently has remained higher since then (Berg, 2010. Personal communication based on the supplemental homicide reports, 1976–2005). Thus, African American and not Caucasian youth in the last two decades have increasingly been drawn into homicide offending and victimization.

In Chap. 3 of this volume, we will see that those young men in the PYS born between about 1974 and 1977 grew up during a large "crime peak" in the Pittsburgh community, while younger men in the study born about 1980 reached their teenage years after this crime peak. Living under different conditions of community crime were associated with different rates of homicide offending and homicide victimization, with those born about 1974–1977 being more often offenders and more often victims than those who were born about the year 1980.

Studies show that, in general, the ages of homicide offenders and victims are positively correlated, with the peak risk being for 19- to 20-year-old males killing other 19- to 20-year-old males (Snyder & Sickmund, 1999, p. 22). Most Caucasian victims (84%) are killed by Caucasian offenders, and similarly most African American victims (91%) are killed by African American offenders (Federal Bureau of Investigation, 2003, p. 22). Thus, the tragedy of homicide among young African American men is doubled by the fact that most of the youth homicides are intraracial. These national figures are much the same for the rates in the Commonwealth of Pennsylvania and for the participants in the PYS at the local level of Pittsburgh (discussed further in Chap. 3).

Youth homicides in the USA differ from those in Europe in at least two major ways. The level of youth homicide is much higher in the USA (Farrington et al., 2004; Roth, 2009), and it is facilitated to a much greater degree by the availability of hand guns. In the USA, most homicide offenders aged 18–24 killed with a gun; in the peak year of 1993, there were three times as many gun homicides as nongun homicides by this age group (Fox & Zawitz, 2001).

There probably is yet another difference between the USA and Europe in the proportions of different types of homicides. Much has been written about types of homicide offenders (e.g., Heide, 2003; Miethe & Regoeczi, 2004; Roberts, Zgoba, & Shahidullah, 2007), but typically the typologies were based on known offender samples rather than on samples from a community such as ours. We expect that the proportion of homicide offenses resulting from serious mental illness (e.g., paranoia associated with schizophrenia or Antisocial Personality Disorder, or psychopathology) is small across different countries, but the cross-national differences are largest when considering street crime-driven homicides. These are homicides associated with the illegal economy (such as drug dealing and dealing in stolen goods) and conflicts of power (such as gang membership and verbal conflicts). They mainly occur on the streets but also can take place indoors.

A community sample, in contrast to a clinical or institutional sample, is less likely to yield information about homicides arising from relatively rare cases of serious mental illness, but is more informative about street crime-driven homicides. Changes in the rate of street-crime type (rather than homicides caused by mental illness) is usually the major force driving changes in national USA levels of homicide (e.g., Blumstein & Wallman, 2000) and street crime-driven homicides constitute the bulk of the homicides reviewed in this volume. We also want to find out to what extent street crime-driven homicide offenders suffer from mental illness (summarized in Chap. 10). Later we will return to the important topic of different categories of homicide offenders.

The Scientific Investigation of the Causes of Homicide Offenders, Violent Offenders, and Their Victims

There are many studies on youth homicide offending, but most of these are very restricted in scope and provide more information about prevalence than about causes. The studies are often good in providing information on how often homicides committed by young people varied nationally over decades (Federal Bureau of Investigation, 2003) and at the local level (Costantino, Kuller, Perper, & Cypess, 1977; Dalton, 2007 Unpublished data). There is also a substantial body of knowledge on the lives of individual homicide offenders (Heide, 1999). However, almost all life history studies of young homicide offenders are based on arrest or court records only (e.g., Wolfgang, 1958), or on a combination of existing records and retrospectively collected information. Homicide studies based on the past self-reported delinquency as well are, as far as we know, not known other than the PYS research reported in this volume.[1]

Outside research studies, much information about youth homicide in judicial proceedings centers around "judicial enquiry and establishing guilt rather than on understanding causal factors" (Hardwick & Rowton-Lee, 1996, p. 273). There has been a great deal of research on the characteristics of young homicide offenders (Heide, 2003), but according to Heide (2004) most such research has been descriptive rather than predictive. We are of the opinion that, because of the way that data are available and used, descriptive research generally has not convincingly established plausible causal factors.

Typically, most descriptive homicide studies have relied on retrospective information about putative causes of homicide. Several problems exist, however, with

---

[1] It should be noted that self-reports of homicide in the PYS were very rare (only two cases).

retrospective life course studies of homicide offenders and victims (Goodman et al., 1988). Court records often provide incomplete information about possible risk factors. Heide (2003, p. 25) pointed out that: "The available literature on youth homicide offenders is retrospective in nature. Retrospective reports by family members are often biased by knowledge that the person has committed an offense, and may be characterized by incomplete or inaccurate recall of critical events and risk factors." The same applies to reports of homicide victims.

This volume differs from other books in several major ways. Prior books and articles on youth homicide mostly dealt with individual case studies based on information collected *after* the homicide had taken place, or with after-the-fact comparisons between groups of homicide offenders and matched controls (e.g., Bailey, 1996; Busch, Zagar, Hughes, Arbit, & Bussell, 1990). This book follows up boys for many years *before* any of them became homicide offenders or homicide victims.

Retrospective case–control studies summarized by Heide (2003) show that homicide offenders tend to come from broken homes and violent families, to have experienced parental alcoholism and child abuse, to have low school achievement, and to have run away from home, truanted, and been suspended from school. Not surprisingly, they also tended to have prior arrest histories.

Methods of studying homicide offenders and victims can be vastly improved when prospective longitudinal surveys are used instead of cross-sectional or retrospective data. Longitudinal surveys based on regular follow-ups of the same individuals over time from childhood into adulthood, preferably based on large community samples, are the best method of establishing causal factors associated with youth murder. The data presented in this book from the PYS show how prospective longitudinal surveys can provide key information about the causes of homicide offending and the causes of homicide victimization.

Current knowledge about the causes of youth homicide offending and violence defies commonly held notions that there is a single major cause. Studies show that there is no single risk factor that can adequately predict violence among young offenders (e.g., Farrington, 2001a; Loeber, Farrington, Stouthamer-Loeber, & White 2008; Loeber et al., 2005a). It is now generally accepted that the probability of individuals committing homicide or violence is enhanced by their exposure to a wide range and an accumulation over time of different risk factors (Heide, 1999). However, past studies differ in the types of risk factors that are identified.

Heide (1999), for example, highlighted family factors (such as child abuse and child neglect), societal influences (such as witnessing violence), resource availability (such as access to guns, involvement with substances), and personal characteristics (such as poor judgment, inability to deal with strong negative feelings). Lewis et al. (1985) in a clinic-referred population identified four main factors: violent fathers, the offender's seizures, psychiatrically hospitalized mothers, and suicidal tendencies. Other researchers have focused on other sets of risk factors (Bender, 1959; Busch, Zagar, Hughes, Arbit, & Bussell, 1990). Typically, researchers often failed to use an inter-disciplinary approach, despite the fact that different factors investigated by different disciplines (e.g., psychiatric illness or neighborhood influences) may all be important in the explanation and prediction of homicide offending (Heide, 1999).

The above questions also apply to the study of the factors predicting homicide victimization. However, there are far fewer homicide victimization studies than homicide offender studies.

The prediction of homicide offenders, violent offenders or victims of homicide, and violence has requirements that are usually absent in most scientific studies to date. First, for an event to qualify as a predictor, it has to occur temporally prior to the offending or the victimization. Second, the study of predictors of offending and victimization becomes more valuable when predictors are compared in a single prediction equation. Only then can one determine what are strongest predictors and which predictors are independent (read: nonoverlapping) of other predictors.

As mentioned, the great majority of homicide offending studies use retrospectively matched controls, which means that putative predictors are not assessed on individuals who may have been similar to homicide offenders at a younger age, but who did not kill anyone. The same problem applies to predictors of homicide victimization. From such studies, we cannot specify the prospective probability of becoming a homicide offender (or victim) for those who possess or do not possess specific risk factors. Such information is essential, because without it we cannot say how well a risk factor works in the prediction of homicide offending or victimization.

Another major limitation of past studies is the fact that homicide offenders and homicide victims are quite rare (typically, less than 5% of samples are offenders or victims). This means that it is much easier to predict that no one will commit homicide (or be murdered) rather than to identify the tiny percentages who are murderers or murdered. Thus, for a prediction study to become really informative, it may be necessary to devise a special prediction tool to overcome the low prevalence of homicide offenders and victims in populations. This is the aim of Chap. 5 (discussed below more in detail).

The present volume addresses the following questions about homicide offenders in the PYS:

- How common are homicides in Pittsburgh, and how does this compare regionally and nationally? (Chap. 3)
- How representative are homicide offenders in the PYS compared to homicide offenders in Allegheny County (where Pittsburgh is located), Pennsylvania, and the USA? (Chap. 3)
- What is the most common type of homicide offender in this study? (Chap. 3)
- What are the circumstances surrounding the homicide crimes, motives of offenders, and weapons used? (Chaps. 3 and 7)

We also address the following questions about prior criminal history, development and prediction of homicide offenders:

- To what extent did homicide offenders engage in antisocial and delinquent behavior earlier in life? (Chaps. 4, 5, and 7)
- Which explanatory, behavioral and criminal risk factors predict homicide offenders out of a community sample up to 22 years later? (Chaps. 4 and 5)
- To what extent can convicted homicide offenders be predicted based on a combination of explanatory, behavioral, and criminal risk factors? (Chaps. 4 and 5)

- Is the prediction of homicide offenders more efficient when based on those who were violent earlier in life compared to a prediction based on the general population of youth? (Chaps. 4 and 5)
- Is there a dose–response relationship between the number of risk factors and the probability of becoming a homicide offender? (Chaps. 4 and 5)
- Do predictors recorded in childhood continue to predict convicted homicide offenders even when predictors recorded in adolescence are taken into account? (Chap. 5)
- Are homicide offenders predominantly psychopaths? (Chaps. 4, 5, and 7)

In the following chapters, most of the above questions will also be addressed for violent boys. In addition, we will address the question:

- How well do risk factors measured during childhood and adolescence predict violence? (Chap. 5)
- Are predictors of homicide offenders qualitatively different from predictors of violent individuals? (Chap. 5)

Types of Homicide Offenders

Not all homicides are the same: they may differ in terms of victim type (such as relative, friend, stranger), motivation (such as conflict, robbery, revenge and retaliation, drug deal gone badly), setting (street gang, school, home), and mental illness (such as antisocial personality, paranoia). For example, Cornell, Benedek, and Benedek (1987) classified youth homicide offenders into three types: psychotic, conflict, and crime (such as robbery). In addition, some researchers have proposed that some offenders are overcontrolled rather than impulsive and undercontrolled (e.g., Hardwick & Rowton-Lee, 1996), but many other typologies have been proposed (e.g., Bijleveld & Smit, 2006; Roberts, Zgoba, & Shahidullah, 2007).

We can expect that the presence of these categories varies in different populations. Fully fledged psychotic conditions are likely to be more present in adulthood than in adolescence or at an earlier age. Psychotic conditions tend to be less common than young homicide offenders (American Psychiatric Association, 1994), which means that there are more young homicide offenders who are not psychotic than psychotic. Similarly, we expect that mental illnesses such as Antisocial Personality Disorder are not very common in inner-city samples characterized by concentrations of poverty and unemployment and other aggregations of risk factors associated with violence. In addition, we expect that undercontrolled young homicide offenders are more typical than overcontrolled young homicide offenders. Heide (1999) in her review of the "profile" of juvenile homicide offenders concluded that:

> today's young killer tends to be male who is unlikely to be psychotic or mentally retarded, to do well in school, or to come from a home in which his biological parents live together in a healthy and peaceful relationship. Rather, he is likely to have experienced or been

exposed to violence in the home and to have a prior arrest record. He is increasingly more likely to use or abuse drugs and alcohol as compared to juvenile homicide offenders of the past (p. 33).

Turning to conflict, we expect that, particularly in the most disadvantaged neighborhoods, there will be more illegal activities (such as drug dealing) which can generate conflicts in which parties apply personal justice rather than seeking the assistance or sanctuary of the police. This means that a higher proportion of conflicts in these areas are going to be settled by angry individuals, who in these areas will have greater access to guns. We expect that homicide offenders will be characterized at a young age by a diagnosis of Disruptive Behavior Disorder, which includes symptoms of aggression and property crime.

It is likely that individuals with disruptive behavior or a high antisocial potential, compared to those with a low antisocial potential, will tend to gravitate to deprived areas and thus become involved in both illegal activities and associated conflict with others. Often, these antisocial individuals, either by choice or because of pervasive unemployment, will engage in illegal economic crime involving drug dealing, selling of stolen goods, and robbing others for money. More of the potential victims of robbery, especially drug dealers, in these settings will be armed. Thus, both selection effects and the effects of known risk factors will converge and make it more likely that antisocial individuals in these settings will get into armed conflict with others, increasing the likelihood that one or more of the combatants will die.

In short, we expect that that the majority of young homicide offenders will not be characterized by mental illnesses, will be highly antisocial when young, will have a long history of undercontrolled behavior, will tend to carry guns, and will engage in illegal activities such as robbery, drug dealing, and gang activity.

Persons Arrested for Homicide but Not Convicted

It may seem a truism that only a proportion of all individuals arrested for homicide will be convicted for homicide. There are several reasons for this. Some individuals suspected of homicide are arrested but are released because their innocence is proved. Others may be brought to court but then released, because of lack of evidence but not necessarily because they are exonerated. Potential witnesses may be terrorized so that they are too frightened to give evidence in court. Much depends on the availability of high-quality evidence, the thoroughness of investigative detective work, and restrictions on the availability of evidence because of, for example, intimidation of witnesses, successful cover-ups, and artful alibis. Also, individuals may have contributed to murder, but may not be held legally responsible; often juries require a higher standard of evidence when judging a potential homicide offender than in other cases.

Even though it is often impossible to state which of the above reasons (or other reasons) apply to individuals arrested for homicide but subsequently not convicted, we believe that that it is worthwhile to examine the characteristics of this group of individuals. First, it is important to know whether arrested but not convicted individuals show a behavioral profile that is very different from convicted homicide offenders, or whether they indeed resemble convicted homicide offenders. To the extent that arrested offenders are truly guilty, they should be similar to convicted offenders; to the extent that arrested offenders are truly innocent, they should be different from convicted offenders. Second, it is of interest to know whether risk factors applicable to homicide offenders also apply to arrested but not convicted individuals. Another argument is that convicted homicide offenders are a biased sample of all homicide offenders, and that arrested plus convicted offenders are a more representative sample. Chapter 4 addresses the following question concerning homicide arrestees who were not convicted for homicide:

- To what extent were the homicide arrestees exposed to the same childhood risk factors as the convicted homicide offenders? (Chap. 4)
- What are the best predictors of the convicted plus arrested homicide offenders (out of all violent boys)? How do these differ from the strongest predictors of the convicted homicide offenders? (Chap. 5)

Homicide Victims

Compared to the number of studies on young homicide offenders, there are relatively few studies on young homicide victims (Ezell & Tanner-Smith, 2009; Lauritsen, Laub, & Sampson, 1992). Homicide victims often feature in official statistics (e.g., Harms & Snyder, 2004), showing that mortality is highest among delinquent populations. For example, Teplin and colleagues (2005) followed up a large sample of youth who had been enrolled in a juvenile justice project. Data on deaths and causes of death were obtained from reports by family members or official records. Out of the total sample, 3.4% died because of homicide, and the mortality rate (deaths per 100,000 person-years) was more than four times greater than in the general population of juveniles of a similar age. The authors concluded that there was a need to study victimization in low- and high-risk populations and to examine risk factors for homicide victimization. Although this would be immensely useful, there is also a need to examine homicide victimization in general populations, particularly in inner-cities where crime is often high. Such studies permit, in a similar fashion to homicide offender studies in the general population, the study of early predictors of homicide victims.

It is also possible to determine the extent to which homicide offenders and homicide victims differ in their earlier behavioral development and their exposure to known risk factors associated with violence. The key question is what the predictors of homicide victimization are, and to what extent these predictors are similar to or different from predictors of homicide offenders. A few studies have compared homicide offenders with victims of homicide (e.g., Brodie, Daday, Crandall, Sklar, & Jost, 2006) showing that homicide offenders and homicide victims are drawn from the same population with similar life experiences. Other studies confirm that assault victims disproportionally tend to have committed violent offenses themselves (e.g., Rivara, Shepherd, Farrington, Richmond, & Cannon, 1995). When combatants are armed with guns and get into a confrontation, who dies may depend on factors such as accuracy of marksmanship, caliber of weapon, or on chance factors. If so, homicide offenders should be quite similar to homicide victims in early risk factors. However, other homicide victims may be more innocent, perhaps in the wrong place at the wrong time and caught in cross-fire.

What we said about the difference between understanding the causes of homicide offending and the prediction of homicide offending also applies to understanding the causes of homicidal victimization and the prediction of homicide victimization. There is much speculation about the causes of homicide victimization. However, to the best of our knowledge, there is a scarcity of studies on the prediction of homicidal victimization outside of intimate relationships (Ezell & Tanner-Smith, 2009). Also, we have not been able to discover validated screening instruments designed to identify youth at risk of violent victimization. For these reasons, this volume addresses both the prediction of homicide victimization and possible ways to screen young males at risk of becoming a victim of homicide.

We will address the following questions concerning homicide victims:

- How common are homicide victims in Pittsburgh? (Chap. 6)
- To what extent did homicide victims engage in antisocial and delinquent behaviors before they were killed? (Chap. 6)
- Which explanatory, behavioral, and criminal risk factors predict homicide victims out of a community sample up to 22 years later? (Chap. 6)
- Is there a dose–response relationship between the number of risk factors and the probability of becoming a homicide victim? (Chap. 6)
- To what extent can homicide victims be predicted based on a combination of explanatory, behavioral, and criminal risk factors? (Chap. 6)

In addition, we will compare homicide offenders and homicide victims and address the following questions:

- Are homicide offenders and victims similar in their antisocial behavior? (Chap. 6)
- Did homicide offenders, compared to homicide victims, grow up under more deprived conditions or were they exposed to more risk factors? (Chap. 6)
- Do early risk factors predict homicide offenders more accurately than homicide victims? (Chap. 6)

Shooting Victims

Most attempts to murder in the USA are committed with hand guns (Roth, 2009), and more people survive than die. Thus, there is a good reason to study shooting victims as well, because they may be similar to homicide victims in terms of their criminal careers. Likewise, the homicide and shooting victims may share many of the known risk factors and may be similar in their prior contacts with the justice system. Thus, as well as comparing homicide victims with homicide offenders, we will also compare homicide victims with the larger group of shooting victims who did not die. We will address the same set as questions for shooting victims that we addressed for homicide victims. In addition, we will ask the following questions:

- Are homicide victims and shooting victims similar in their antisocial behavior? (Chap. 6)
- Do early risk factors predict homicide victims more accurately than shooting victims? (Chap. 6)

Screening

Prediction data are the building blocks for the construction of screening devices to identify youth at risk. We are interested in finding out to what extent it is possible to screen for homicide offenders and victims of homicide at a young age. Much has been written about screening instruments to identify violent offenders (see Conroy & Murrie, 2007, who in Chap. 7 review risk assessments with juvenile offenders; Webster & Hucker, 2007), but most of the instruments have been validated on adult populations after incarceration. The few screening instruments for younger individuals focus on the risk of later problem behavior (e.g., the EARL-20B developed by Augimeri, Koegl, Webster, & Levene, 2001), and only one specifically assesses the risk of violence in populations of juvenile offenders (the SAVRY developed by Borum, Bartel, & Forth, 2006). We are not aware of any screening instrument designed to identify juvenile victims of violence.

The common requirements of all screening devices are that the instruments: (a) perform better than chance and (b) have low error rates. A distinction has been made between false-positive errors (identifying someone at risk for violence who does not become violent) and false-negative errors (identifying someone as not at risk for violence who does become violent). It is our opinion, that for serious outcomes such as homicide offending and victimization, it is most important to minimize false-negative rather than false-positive errors because of the major consequences attached to losing a life. However, at the same time, a high proportion of false-positive errors is undesirable because they can overload intervention programs to reduce violence and can be very costly.

Screening instruments to identify youth at risk for homicide offending or homicide victimization can be used for different age groups. However, it is generally recognized that false-positive and false-negative errors vary with the age of screening. It is often thought that false-positive errors are high for screening devices applied to preschool populations because many children at that age show age-normative disruptive behaviors (e.g., temper tantrums) that they tend to outgrow later. On the other hand, scholars have proposed that many of the most serious offenders start their delinquency careers early in life (e.g., Farrington, 1996; Farrington & Loeber, 2000a; Loeber & Farrington 2001; Moffitt, 1993), which argues for screening at a younger rather than an older age. In another line of reasoning, we would expect that, at some point in development, screening at a later age, say in adolescence, would become less efficient because of a preponderance of false-negative errors, resulting from the screening instrument not capturing future homicide offenders because they have already become violent at a young age. Briefly, we propose that screening for homicide risk at say age 7 is better than at age 13 (because of lower false-negative errors), but it is an open question whether this applies to homicide victimization as well. We address screening issues and instruments in Chaps. 4–6.

There is another, underutilized way of approaching screening, which fits the much advocated notion that there should be a link between risk assessment and risk management (e.g., Ireland, Ireland, & Birch, 2009). Briefly, the arguments behind it are as follows. Conventional screening is aimed at the identification of deviant individuals before deviancy becomes manifest. Interventions are another major tool to address the optimal age of identification of at-risk groups. Preventive interventions are aimed at steering youth away from a life of crime, including from becoming a homicide offender or a homicide victim.

The following chapters address several key questions relevant to the early screening of individuals at risk for homicide offending or victimization:

- To what extent is it possible to develop and use a screening instrument to predict persons who are at risk of becoming homicide offenders or victims? (Chap. 10)
- Is a step-wise screen more efficient in the prediction of homicide offenders compared to a single screen? (Chap. 5)
- Is it possible to model screening and establish whether an early screen is more efficient in identifying homicide offenders than a screen administered at a later age? (Chaps. 8 and 9)
- Is a screening instrument for the prediction of homicide offenders better or worse than a screening instrument for the prediction of homicide victims? (Chap. 10)

The Issue of Race

As mentioned, studies show that African American males are overrepresented among homicide offenders and homicide victims (e.g., Pope & Snyder, 2003; Strom & MacDonald, 2007). The increase in homicide offending that took place in the early 1990s was largely driven by an increase in homicides by and of African American males (Harms & Snyder, 2004). In the Pittsburgh Youth Study, the majority of the violent offenders and homicide offenders were African American (Farrington, Loeber, & Stouthamer-Loeber, 2003), and so were the homicide victims (Farrington et al., 2003; Loeber et al., 1999b). Yet, we found that African American race did not predict violent offenders in multivariate analyses after controlling for other risk factors (Loeber et al., 2008). This shows that African American race is a predictor primarily because it is associated with risk factors such as broken families and living in the worst, most deprived neighborhoods. It is not clear, however, whether this also applies at a young age. The following questions will be addressed:

- Are racial differences in the prevalence of violent and homicide offenders attributable to racial differences in early risk factors? (Chaps. 4 and 5)

- Are racial differences in the prevalence of homicide and shooting victims attributable to racial differences in early risk factors? (Chap. 9)

Theories About Homicide Offenders and Homicide Victims

Most people have some idea about the causes of homicide offending and might think of mental illness, poor rearing conditions in families, deprived neighborhoods, and so on, as possible causes. Homicide and violence reports overflow with myths, theories, and loose ideas about which causes are truly important in the commission of homicide offending and violence (but see reviews by Farrington, 2005, in press; Heide, 1999; Thornberry & Krohn, 2003). For centuries, the verifiability of these notions has been frustratingly difficult.

Increasingly, criminologists have formulated interconnected ideas (also called theories) to explain delinquency in general and violence in particular (see, e.g., chapters in Farrington, 2005). Invariably the theories put emphasis on some rather than other explanations, which tend to vary over individual (including biological), family, peer, and neighborhood influences. Theories also tend to differ in the extent to which they emphasize proximal factors (e.g., routine activities) in comparison to more distal factors (e.g., parents' early childrearing deficiencies). For example, Farrington (2005, Chap. 4) formulated an integrated cognitive antisocial potential theory which includes short-term and long-term factors, mostly based on results from many different studies (discussed more in detail in Chap. 10). The factors include various forms of deprivation (e.g., low income), criminality of parents or peers, living in a disadvantaged neighborhood, poor childrearing practices by parents, antisocial potential and impulsivity of the youth, exposure to known risk factors including stressful life events, opportunities for offending and victimization in the context of routine activities, and decision-making processes. The theory also recognizes that offending may have several negative consequences that further increase the probability of offending.

Most delinquency theories assume that there is no need to have a specific explanation of homicide offending, but do not address whether homicide offenders are similar to other violent offenders who have not committed homicide. Theories also tend to differ in major ways in the extent to which they are inspired by and/or supported by empirical findings. Thus, for the scientific study of homicide to proceed, we need to be able to establish the predictive accuracy of certain variables and determine whether there are quantitative or qualitative differences between homicide offenders and nonhomicidal violent offenders. It is also important to demonstrate that some risk factors predicted homicide offenders and victims after controlling for other risk factors. A quantitative difference would apply when homicide offenders share risk factors with those who are violent but not homicidal, but homicide offenders score higher than nonhomicidal violent offenders on those risk factors, or possess more risk factors. In contrast, there would be a qualitative difference if homicide offenders were characterized by different risk factors from nonhomicidal violent offenders.

Another approach to causality is to ask homicide offenders about why they committed a homicide (detailed in Chap. 7). The advantage of such an approach is that it reveals causal influences that are more proximal to the actual homicide event. However, homicide offenders may not be truthful about the circumstances that led up the homicide, particularly when they are awaiting sentencing, and they may not fully understand the factors that influenced their behavior. Also, homicide victims cannot be questioned about their crimes (detailed in Chap. 7).

Property crime, violence, and the illegal economy. In the course of this volume we confirm something that has been known for many years, that offending and victimization are intertwined with often the same individuals being offenders and becoming victims (e.g., Brodie, Daday, Crandall, Sklar, & Jost, 2006; Ezell & Tanner-Smith, 2009; Lauritsen, Sampson, & Laub, 1991). Often the notion prevails that what connects violent offenders and their victims is that "violence begets violence." This certainly can be the case. However, what we want to explore in this volume is whether homicide offenders and violent offenders on one hand, and homicide victims and shooting victims on the other hand, share many aspects of their development, are exposed to similar risk factors (see Chaps. 4–6), and engage in high-risk forms of *property crime*. Whereas drug selling is often thought to be an example of such behavior, we will also investigate the role of other property crimes, such as receiving and selling stolen goods, car theft, and theft from a car as the most important examples. Thus, we propose that these illegal forms of property crime attract aggressive individuals (a selection effect), and that the nature of the illegal property transactions generates conflict which, in an atmosphere of nonreporting of crime to the police, are resolved outside the law by means of the administration of "personal justice."

Turning to theories of victimization, most delinquency theories are silent on explanations of why some individuals become victims of homicide or violence (see, e.g., Farrington, 2005).

In summary, we will address the following questions about theories concerning homicide offenders and homicide victims and their policy implications:

- On the basis of the empirical findings, which criminological theories best explain the development of young homicide offenders and victims? (Chap. 10)
- How can current policies to reduce youth violence and homicide offending be optimized? (Chap. 10)

Incarceration vs. Prevention

Much of the debate about what to do to reduce homicide rates locally and nationally focuses on sentencing of offenders, especially in terms of long-term incarceration and absence of or restrictions on early release and parole (Spelman, 2000). Part of this debate is not just a question of the administration of just deserts, but it has to do with the protection of citizens in the open society from revictimization by known dangerous offenders. Overall, this debate has centered on retribution and is not necessarily driven by knowledge about homicide offenders, such as whether the majority of these offenders are one-time homicide offenders rather than serial killers (which are rare). Also, since the prevalence of homicide offending (and violence) peaks in late adolescence and early adulthood, it is likely that a high proportion of homicide offenders will desist from further violence in their 20s. More information is needed about recidivism rates. A second issue concerns the alleged mental imbalance of homicide offenders. Particularly, the media often depict them as unpredictable psychopaths, whose behavior is governed by impulsive personality traits that are thought to be stable over time.

It is worthwhile to judge several arguments against this grim picture of homicide offenders. Some individuals argue that killers are made rather than born and that they develop over time on a pathway of gradually increasing severity of aggressive and violent acts that eventually culminate in homicide (Loeber et al., 2005). We know from several studies that homicidal and violent offenders are exposed to a variety of criminogenic factors, including having been poorly reared, many changes in caretakers, poor school success, affiliation with delinquent peers, and living in very disadvantaged neighborhoods characterized by a low prevalence of protective factors (e.g., Loeber et al., 2005).

Earlier homicide studies have occasionally referred to the need to prevent homicide by reducing known risk factors (e.g., Heide, 2003). However, we are not aware of intervention studies that have had homicide offending or homicide victimization as outcome measures. We think that this largely reflects the low numbers of homicide offenders and homicide victims in research samples, the low prevalence of both outcomes in the general population and the relatively short follow-up of treated and control samples in most intervention studies. Our assumption is that interventions addressing the causes of violence will also address the causes of homicide offending and homicide victimization.

Scholars who are aware of the accumulation of risk factors in the lives of certain individuals often conclude that society's answer to violence and homicide should not be restricted to long-term incarceration but should also focus on prevention. In this volume, we will present data showing to what extent homicide offending can be predicted and which of the predictors are potentially modifiable. Second, we will use simulation studies to demonstrate to what extent known interventions may reduce homicide offending in the foreseeable future (Chaps. 8 and 9). In this way, we hope that we can extend the debate on the prevention of violence to the reduction of homicide offending and, indirectly, homicide victimization.

The simulation work can also address the key question of whether intervention at an early age produces a better outcome (more violence prevented, including homicide offending and homicide victimization, and a lower rate of incarceration) than intervention at a later age. We are not aware of intervention studies that have systematically investigated what is the optimal age of intervention to reduce future homicide offending or homicide victimization.

We will address the following questions pertaining to the model of the impact of interventions at the national level:

- When modeling nationwide interventions focused on high-risk youth, how much decrease in the national homicide rate can we expect? (Chap. 8)
- Is early intervention more efficient than later intervention? (Chap. 9)

The next set of questions concerns the modeling of the impact of interventions at a local level:

- To what extent does an intervention with a success rate of 30% that focuses on high-risk boys at a young age (ages 10–13; Screen 1) reduce arrests for violence as shown in the age–crime curve, and other indicators of violent offending and incarceration? (Chap. 9)
- Does an intervention at age 14 only based on arrest for violence have sufficient benefits if an intervention already has taken place at an earlier age? (Chap. 9)
- What is the yield of an intervention at age 14 based on arrest for violence without an intervention at an earlier age? (Chap. 9)
- How well do the two interventions compare when serious delinquency is the outcome? (Chap. 9)
- Does an intervention at a young age have a higher yield in reducing the frequency of serious delinquency than an intervention at age 13? (Chap. 9)

The Goals of this Book

This book reports on the prospective prediction of homicide offenders and victims using a wide variety of risk factors in three representative school samples that comprise the PYS. The PYS is a longitudinal investigation of the causes of delinquency in inner-city boys, who have been followed from childhood to early adulthood (Loeber & Farrington, 2001; Loeber et al., 2003; Loeber, Farrington, Stouthamer-Loeber, & van Kammen, 1998; Loeber et al., 2008; see Chap. 2). We provide information about the prevalence of homicide offenders and victims, the circumstances under which homicides were committed, the development and characteristics of offenders and victims, and the extent to which offenders and victims can be predicted by early risk factors.

This volume builds on our earlier publications on homicide offenders and victims in the PYS (Farrington, Loeber, Stallings, & Homish, 2008; Loeber et al., 1999a; Loeber et al., 2005) using updated information on homicide offenders and victims up to May 2009. The volume is also inspired by a major set of longitudinal analyses on violence in general committed by young males in the same study (Loeber et al., 2008). In summary, the present volume, in comparison with past PYS research, is based on larger samples of offenders and victims, and addresses a host of new questions to shed new light on homicide offenders, homicide arrestees, homicide victims, and shooting victims.

Chapter 2
The Pittsburgh Youth Study

Rolf Loeber, David P. Farrington, and Rebecca Stallings

This chapter reviews the design and data collection procedures of the Pittsburgh Youth Study (PYS). It builds on the first book on the PYS, which focused on the first two waves of the study (Loeber, Farrington, Stouthamer-Loeber, & van Kammen 1998a), and on the second book of the PYS (Loeber, Farrington, Stouthamer-Loeber, & White, 2008), which covers all available data waves for the youngest and oldest cohorts between ages 7 and 25.

Pittsburgh. Pittsburgh is largely a blue-collar city, formerly dominated by the steel industry. It is situated in the confluence of two rivers (see Fig. 3.4 in Chap. 3), which join to form the Ohio River. In the 2000 Census (the year in which the young males were between 20 and 26 years old), the Pittsburgh metropolitan area had about 2,358,695 inhabitants and the City of Pittsburgh had about 334,563 citizens, of which 26% were African American, 72% Caucasian, and the remainder (2%) were from other ethnic groups. In 2000, the city counted 18,612 boys between ages 0 and 9, 15,220 boys between ages 10 and 17, and 24,742 young men between ages 18 and 24.

Pittsburgh has a very stable population; 80% of the residents had been born in the state, compared to 62% on average across the USA. Only 3% of Pittsburgh inhabitants were foreign born compared to 8% across the USA and only 2% of the City's population was not fluent in English. The median family income in Pittsburgh was similar to that in the USA as a whole, with 17% of the children living below the poverty level. There are 90 neighborhoods in the city, many of which, because of rivers, railways, or ravines, are geographically distinct. Most of the neighborhoods are racially divided, with African Americans tending to live in the most disadvantaged neighborhoods.

Design. The PYS is a longitudinal study consisting of the repeated follow-ups of community cohorts of inner-city boys, which began in 1987 (for the successive assessments, see Table 2.1). The boys were in grades 1, 4, and 7 in Pittsburgh public schools at the outset of the study (called youngest, middle, and oldest cohorts). With the assistance of the Pittsburgh Board of Education, we started out with comprehensive public school lists of the enrollment of 1,631, 1,432, and 1,419 male students in grades

2 The Pittsburgh Youth Study

Table 2.1 Design and sequence of assessments in the Pittsburgh Youth Study

Youngest cohort (Grade 1 at screening)

Mean age	6.2	6.7	7.2	7.7	8.2	8.7	9.2	9.7	10.2	11	12	13	14	15	16	17	18	19
Wave	S	A	B	C	D	E	F	G	H	J	L	N	P	R	T	V	Y	AA

Middle cohort (Grade 4 at screening)

Mean age	9.5	10	10.5	11	11.5	12	12.5
Wave	S	A	B	C	D	E	F

Oldest cohort (Grade 7 at screening)

Mean age	12.6	13.1	13.6	14.1	14.6	15.1	16	17	18	19	20	21	22	23	24	25
Wave	S	A	B	C	D	E	G	I	K	M	O	Q	SS	U	W	Z

Note: The age shown is the mean age of participants at the midpoint of the 6-month or 1-year period preceding the assessment

1, 4, and 7, respectively. From these lists, we randomly selected about 1,100 boys in each of the three grades to be contacted (1,165, 1,146, and 1,125 in grades 1, 4, and 7, respectively). However, a number of the children had moved out of the school district, proved to be girls, or were of an incorrect age. Eventually, we contacted 1,006, 1,004, and 998 families with eligible boys in grades 1, 4, and 7, respectively.

The participation rate of boys and their parents was 84.6%, 86.3%, and 83.9% of the eligible boys in the youngest, middle, and oldest cohorts, respectively. Because of the high participation rate of families at the beginning of the study, we believe that the cohorts are representative of the populations from which they were drawn, namely boys in grades 1, 4, and 7 in Pittsburgh public schools. A comparison of those who participated and those who did not indicated that there were no significant differences in racial distribution and achievement test results, which were the only two variables that could be compared from school records (Loeber, Farrington et al., 1998). Furthermore, the cohorts are reasonably representative of boys in the general population in the City of Pittsburgh, because 72% of all students residing within the city limits were enrolled in the public schools in 1987 (Loeber, Farrington et al., 1998). Although no figures could be obtained on the differences between public school students and private or parochial school students, it is a reasonable assumption that those students not enrolled in public schools were more likely to be Caucasian and of higher socioeconomic status than the public school students.

Screening. In order to increase the number of high-risk males, we used a screening assessment at wave S. On this basis of this screening, which used information from the participant, his parent, and his teacher, the 30% of the boys identified as the most antisocial were included in the follow-up cohort, together with another 30% who were randomly selected from the remaining 70%. This strategy has the dual advantages of drawing conclusions about the population by weighting the results back to the original population (e.g., Stouthamer-Loeber, Loeber, & Thomas, 1992), while maximizing the yield of deviant outcomes. This resulted in the final cohorts of 503, 508, and 506 boys in grades 1, 4, and 7, respectively, who together with their parent were to be followed up. Table 2.2 summarizes the characteristics of the cohorts, who differed in the age (of course) and in the percentage of students held back.

Table 2.2 Characteristics of the cohorts at the beginning of the study (Wave A; Loeber, Farrington et al., 1998)

	Youngest	Middle	Oldest
Participant			
% African American	57.7	55.9	57.5
>50th Percentile CAT reading score	54.5	37.6	35.2
Average age	6.7	10.0	13.1
% Held back in school	26.3	34.1	39.4
Family			
% Living with natural mother	95.2	92.2	94.0
% Living with natural father	39.6	41.5	37.1
% Not living with (acting) father	45.7	40.6	45.3
% (Acting) mother not completed high school	17.3	18.8	19.6
% (Acting) mother with college degree	6.3	5.7	7.4
% (Acting) father not completed high school	16.9	16.2	20.4
% (Acting) father with college degree	12.4	11.7	10.4

Note: Numbers may slightly differ from earlier publications because of later recleaning of data

Extent of the Follow-Ups. The youngest cohort (*N* = 503) has been assessed a total of 18 consecutive times from middle childhood to late adolescence (from age 6 to 19), while the oldest cohort (*N* = 506) has been assessed a total of 16 consecutive times from early adolescence to early adulthood (from age 13 to 25).[1] Assessments of each of the cohorts were carried out initially half-yearly (nine assessments for the youngest cohort and six assessments for the oldest cohort), and later yearly (see Table 2.1). Each of the assessment intervals was contiguous (in other words, without gaps), which meant that the study is uniquely poised to investigate individuals' onset of delinquency and substance use, and individuals' continuation of and desistance from these behaviors. The middle cohort (*N* = 508) was only assessed seven times, at half-yearly intervals from age 10 to 13.

Developmental Pathways to Violence

The media and lay people often perceive homicide and other types of violence (aggravated assault, robbery, and forcible rape) as events that are committed by psychopaths whose behavior has the added edge of unpredictability. Another view, however, is that homicide and violence are the culmination of a gradual developmental process taking place over many years. The assumption is that homicide and violence in some ways are predictable and that they are most likely to take place if

---

[1] The youngest cohort was later followed up in the mid-20s, and that cohort and the oldest cohort are currently (2010–2011) being followed up at about ages 30 and 36, respectively.

aggressive patterns of behavior (other than violence and homicide offending) are present earlier in life. To find out more about such sequences of aggression, researchers have studied developmental pathways to serious delinquency and violence.

There is now a body of research findings on developmental pathways to violence. Research initially based on the PYS showed evidence for three pathways, one of which is relevant for violence. These are the overt, covert, and authority conflict pathways (Loeber, DeLamatre, Keenan, & Zhang, 1998b; Loeber, Wei, Stouthamer-Loeber, Huizinga, & Thornberry, 1999; Loeber et al., 1993). Youths typically follow a remarkably orderly progression from less to more serious antisocial behaviors from childhood to adolescence (Loeber, Keenan, & Zhang, 1997; Loeber et al., 1993). Particularly relevant for this volume is the overt pathway that starts with minor aggression, has physical fighting as a second stage, and more serious violence as a third stage.

The pathways model has been validated in the Denver and Rochester samples (Loeber, Wei et al., 1999) and also in the Chicago Youth Development Study and the National Youth Survey. Tolan, Gorman-Smith, and Loeber (2000) replicated the triple-pathway model in a sample of African American and Hispanic adolescents in Chicago and in a nationally representative US sample of adolescents. The pathways model also reflects selection processes in that increasingly smaller groups of youth are at risk for the more serious behaviors, comparable to a successive sieving process. A key issue for this volume is the extent to which homicide offenders emerge from the group of violent boys, or whether the majority of homicide offenders emerge from boys who were nonviolent boys at a younger age.

Recent research on homicide has expanded the overt pathway model. We propose that homicide is the culmination of prior violence and that the majority of homicide offenders, prior to the commission of homicide, were known for their violence. Research in the PYS showed that this was indeed the case: almost all homicide offenders (95%) had committed violence prior to committing the homicide (Loeber et al., 2005a).

Other Findings on Violence

The PYS has generated a wealth of findings on violence (aggravated assault, robbery, and forcible rape) that are relevant for understanding homicide as a specific form of violence. The following are examples of findings on violence in the PYS to date.

Development and Course. We will concentrate on physical fighting and violence since the former tends to be a precursor to the latter. The stability of physical aggression tends to increase between ages 6–7 and 9–10 (Loeber & Hay, 1997), well prior to adolescence. However, research shows that the prevalence of aggression, including physical aggression, tends to decrease between childhood and adolescence. This reflects the fact that there are normative changes in aggression with a proportion of aggressive individuals outgrowing physical fighting and verbal aggression. However, a minority of aggressive juveniles does not de-escalate, but becomes worse in that they start to engage in more violent acts, such as robbery, rape, and aggravated assault (Loeber & Hay, 1997; Loeber et al., 2008).

Violence and Serious Theft. Whereas serious theft and violence other than homicide appear to be more common in the early part of criminal careers (ages 13–16), homicide tend to occur later (Loeber et al., 2008; see also Chap. 3). We also found that the persistence of violence is higher than that of serious theft. This implies that desistance from serious theft tends to occur earlier than desistance from violence (Loeber et al., 2008).

Secular Changes. Violence in societies tends to fluctuate across the years and tends to peak in some years and be lower in other years (called secular changes). This means that the proportion of each generation who becomes violent is not constant, but varies over the decades. In the Pittsburgh Youth Study, we found (Loeber et al., 2008) that the oldest cohort was much more violent than the youngest cohort. Even though the cohorts were only 6 years apart, the oldest cohort engaged more in serious forms of delinquency such as gang membership and drug dealing, which often are associated with violence.

We mentioned a developmental pathway of aggression in which physical fighting is the second step and violence is the third step. The question is to what extent secular changes in aggression are reflected in developmental pathways. Is the probability of escalation from physical fighting to violence different from generation to generation, or is the prevalence of physical fighting different among different age cohorts, which would explain why a larger proportion of young men escalate to violence (and homicide offending) in one generation compared to another? Findings from the PYS indicate that the probability of escalation from physical fighting to violence was the same for the youngest and oldest cohorts, but what differed between the cohorts was the proportion of physical fighters, which was higher in the oldest compared to the youngest cohort. A comparison between two cohorts, however, is only limited evidence that secular changes in violence can be predicted by secular changes in physical fighting, which can be measured years before the eruption of violence.

Generations of youth also differ in the rate at which they outgrow violence in late adolescence and early adulthood. The outgrowing processes occurred quicker for the youngest compared to the oldest cohort (Loeber et al., 2008). This implies that the youngest cohort's bout with physically victimizing others was of shorter duration, and hence involved fewer victims and incidents of victimization.

Associations between Violence and Other Problem Behaviors. Research findings from many studies have shown that problem behaviors often are associated with other problem behaviors (Jessor & Jessor, 1997). People tend to be versatile rather than specialized in their antisocial behavior. However, different types of offenses are not equally linked to violence. For example, in the PYS, we found that hard drug use was related to theft but not to violence, while drug dealing was related to violence but not to theft (Loeber et al., 2008).

Causation. The causes of violence lie in the individual, family, peer group, school, and neighborhood (Loeber et al., 2005a, 2008). There is a dose–response relationship between the number of risk factors to which young males are exposed and the probability of their becoming violent (Loeber et al., 2005a). Most of the risk factors for violence identified in the PYS have also been documented in other longitudinal studies with a variety of populations. For example, explanatory factors for violence in the PYS are similar to explanatory factors for violence in inner-city London (Farrington, 1998; Farrington & Loeber, 1999).

The causes of violence only partly differ from the causes of theft. In the PYS, the strongest predictors of violence were generally similar to the strongest predictors of theft at younger ages, but not at older ages. This indicates that there are many unique factors predictive of violence and unique factors predictive of theft. For example, gun carrying and the family living on welfare were the best predictors of violence, whereas child maltreatment, theft victimization, and Caucasian race were the best predictors of theft (Loeber et al., 2008).

Violence occurs in both disadvantaged and advantaged neighborhoods, but it tends to be concentrated in disadvantaged neighborhoods. The best predictor of repeated violence in advantaged neighborhoods was earlier physical aggression, but the best predictors of repeated violence in disadvantaged neighborhoods were: lack of guilt, having early sex, carrying a hidden weapon, and poor parent–child communication (Beyers, Loeber, Wikström, & Stouthamer-Loeber, 2001). This implies that violence in advantaged neighborhoods may be driven more by individual factors (such as aggression), while violence in disadvantaged neighborhoods is more a function of social- and context-dependent factors.

Race and Violence. Violence is more common in African American than in Caucasian males (Cook & Laub, 1998; Mercy, Rosenberg, Powell, Broome, & Roper, 1993; Snyder & Sickmund, 1995). African American males in the PYS were more likely than Caucasians to be arrested and convicted for violence (Chap. 3). The PYS could not address the extent to which the overrepresentation of African American men in the justice system might have been caused by racial discrimination at the levels of the police, justice intake officers, court personnel, or probation officers. Results from the PYS showed that African American race did not predict reported violence (based on self-reports and information from parents and teachers) once other risk factors (such as bad neighborhood, old for the grade) were taken into account. However, when the analyses were repeated with Court reports of violence as the outcome, African American race contributed to the prediction of violence even when other factors were taken into account (Farrington, Loeber, & Stouthamer-Loeber, 2003). In this volume, we address the issue of whether race predicts homicide offending after controlling for other risk factors.

Measurements and Constructs

This study has a wealth of measurements and constructs based on the measurements. For brevity's sake, the constructs used in this book, the waves in which they were measured, and the measurements on which they have been based are summarized in Table 2.3.

Table 2.3 Description of constructs

Risk factor (respondent)[a] / Source	Instrument[b]	Waves[c]	No. of items[d]	Example questions	Answer Scale or cutoff	Alpha (for scales)[d]
Child behavior factors:						
Screening risk score (PTY) Loeber, Farrington et al. (1998)	Screening: CBCL/YSR, SRA/SRD	S	21	Ever run away, set fires, attack, truancy, gang fight, vandalism, stealing, joyride, hit/hurt teacher or parent, robbery, burglary, arrested, use alcohol, marijuana, sniff glue	Highest 1/3	N/A
Cruel to people (PT) Achenbach and Edelbrock (1979, 1983), Edelbrock and Achenbach (1984)	CBCL, TRF	S and A	4	Cruelty, bullying, meanness to others	3-Point Likert	0.34 (Y) 0.62 (M) 0.57 (O)
Cruel to animals (P) Achenbach and Edelbrock (1979, 1983)	CBCL	S and A	2	Animal cruelty	3-Point Likert	N/A
Depressed mood (Y) Angold, Erkanli, Loeber, Costello, Van Kammen and Stouthamer-Loeber (1996)	Recent Mood and feelings questionnaire	A	13	Over the past two weeks, felt unhappy, hard to concentrate, did everything wrong, did not enjoy anything, felt unloved, tired	3-Point Likert	0.80 (Y) 0.82 (M) 0.84 (O)
Shy/withdrawn (PT) Achenbach and Edelbrock (1979, 1983), Edelbrock and Achenbach (1984)	CBCL, TRF	S and A	14	Likes to be alone, is withdrawn, refuses to talk, self-conscious, shy	3-Point Likert	0.79 (Y) 0.80 (M) 0.83 (O)
Physical aggression (PT) Achenbach and Edelbrock (1979, 1983), Edelbrock and Achenbach (1984)	CBCL, TRF	S and A	29	Getting into fights, physically attacking others, hitting parents or teacher	3-Point Likert	0.87 (Y) 0.89 (M) 0.86 (O)

(continued)

Table 2.3 (continued)

Risk factor (respondent)[a] Source	Instrument[b]	Waves[c]	No. of items[d]	Example questions	Answer Scale or cutoff	Alpha (for scales)[d]
Nonphysical aggression (PT) Achenbach and Edelbrock (1979, 1983), Edelbrock and Achenbach (1984)	CBCL, TRF	S and A	62	Bragging, swearing, demanding attention, defiant or talking back, disobedient, disrupting class, jealous, showing off	3-Point Likert	0.94 (Y) 0.96 (M) 0.95 (O)
Covert behavior (PTY) Loeber, Farrington et al. (1998)	CBCL, TRF, YSR	S and A	50 (Y) 49 (M) 54 (O)	Concealing, untrustworthy, manipulative: Lies/ cheats, Says he is one place when someplace else, cannot trust what he says, when confronted about behavior, is a fast or smooth talker, stays out late at night	3-Point Likert	0.90 (Y) 0.93 (M) 0.93 (O)
Callous/unemotional (T)	TRF	A	14	Teases a lot, does not seem to feel guilty after misbehaving, explosive/unpredictable	3-Point Likert	0.92 (Y) 0.94 (M) 0.95 (O)
Runs away (PY) Loeber, Farrington et al. (1998)	CBCL, SRA/SRD	S and A	2	Runs away from home	3-Point Likert No/yes	
HIA: hyperactivity–impulsivity –attention problems (PT) Loeber, Farrington et al. (1998)	CBCL, TRF	S and A	25	Difficulty concentrating, restless, wants things right away, impulsive, talks too much, trouble following directions	3-Point Likert	0.86 (Y) 0.87 (M) 0.88 (O)
Child attitudes/cognition:						
Positive attitude to substance use (Y) Loeber, Farrington et al. (1998)	Attitude Toward Delinquent Behavior Scale	A	3 (Y) 4 (MO)	How wrong for someone your age to... Sell hard drugs (LSD, cocaine, heroin)? Drink alcohol? Use marijuana, hashish, or pot? Use heroin, cocaine, or LSD?	4-Point Likert	0.50 (Y) 0.84 (M) 0.80 (O)
Unlikely to get caught (Y) Loeber, Farrington et al. (1998)	Likelihood of Being Caught Scale	C (Y) A (MO)	9 (Y) 10 (MO)	How likely do you think it is that you will get caught by police if you... Damage or destroy something? Steal something worth <$5? Hit someone to hurt? Use alcohol?	3-Point Likert	0.70 (Y) 0.91 (M) 0.89 (O)
Low school motivation (T) Loeber, Farrington et al. (1998)	TRF	S and A	2	Compared to typical pupils of the same age. How hard is he working?	7-Point Likert	N/A

Construct (Reference)	Instrument	Informant	No.	Description	Scale
Lack of guilt (PT) Loeber, Farrington et al. (1998)	CBCL, TRF	S and A	2	Does not seem to feel guilty after misbehaving	3-Point Likert
Positive attitude to delinquency (Y) Loeber, Farrington et al. (1998)	Attitude Toward Delinquent Behavior Scale	A	9 (Y) 11 (MO)	How wrong do you think it is for someone your age to skip school? shoplift? damage property? hit an adult? rob with weapon?	4-Point Likert
Child psychiatric diagnoses:					
At least one Disruptive Behavior Diagnosis (P) Loeber, Farrington et al. (1998)	DISC-P	A	3	Meets DSM-IIIR criterion for attention deficit hyperactivity disorder, conduct disorder, or oppositional defiant disorder	
ADHD: Attention Deficit Hyperactivity Disorder (P) Loeber, Farrington et al. (1998)	DISC-P	A	28	Is it almost always hard for him to sit still? Does he find it difficult to finish something you ask him to do? When he has to stand in line, does he often try to push ahead or get in ahead of his turn?	3-Point Likert · Symptom criteria for DSMIII-R diagnosis
CD: Conduct Disorder (P) Loeber, Farrington et al. (1998)	DISC-P	A	13	Has he ever cut school, played hooky, been truant? Does he get into many fist (physical) fights? Has he ever attacked someone and hurt them badly?	3-Point Likert · Symptom criteria for DSMIII-R diagnosis
ODD: Oppositional Defiant Disorder (P) Loeber, Farrington et al. (1998)	DISC-P	A	13	Does he often argue with or talk back to you? Does he often seem to deliberately annoy you or other adults or kids? Does he often swear, use bad language, talk dirty, or use obscene words?	3-Point Likert · Symptom criteria for DSMIII-R diagnosis

(continued)

Table 2.3 (continued)

Risk factor (respondent)[a] / Source	Instrument[b]	Waves[c]	No. of items[d]	Example questions	Answer Scale or cutoff	Alpha (for scales)[d]
Child's history of offending:						
Delinquency seriousness classification (PTY) — Loeber, Farrington et al. (1998)	CBCL, TRF, SRA/ SRD, YSR	S and A		Parent: Carries a weapon. Gang fights Teacher: Uses force or strongarm methods to get money or things Youth: In the past year have you purposely damaged or destroyed something that did not belong to you? Avoided paying for things? Gone into building to steal?	3-Point Likert No/yes	N/A
Carrying weapon – any (PY)	CBCL, SRD	E	4	Parent: Carries a weapon Youth: In the past year, have you carried a hidden weapon?	3-Point Likert No/yes	N/A
Gun carrying (Y)	SRD	S, A-F	1	Thinking of the most serious time you carried a hidden weapon (most dangerous weapon): What kind of weapon was it?	Open-ended	N/A
Weapon use (Y)	SRD	G-P(Y) A-F(M) A-G(O)	3	Used weapon (other than gun) during most serious time you attacked someone, or used force to get things, or gang fight (did either group use weapons)?	No/yes	N/A
Gang membership (Y)	Gang Questionnaire	H-P(Y) D-F(M) D-G(O)	1	Have you ever been a member of a youth or street gang?	No/yes	N/A
Gang fight (PY)	CBCL, SRD	E	2	Caretaker: Gang fights Youth: In the past year have you been in a gang fight?	3-Point Likert No/yes	N/A
Persistent drug use (Y)	Substance Use Scale	G-P(Y) A-F(M) S, A-G(O)	3	Top 25% frequency and severity/type of substance (alcohol, marijuana, hard drugs) for 3+ waves	N/A	

Construct	Instrument	Coding		Question	Response	
Sells marijuana (Y)	SRD	G-P(Y), A-F(M), S, A-G(O)	7	Have you ever/in the past year sold marijuana or hashish?	No/yes	N/A
Sells hard drugs (Y)	SRD	G-P(Y), A-F(M), S, A-G(O)	7	Have you ever/past year sold hard drugs?	No/yes	N/A
Robbery (Y)	SRD	G-P(Y), A-F(M), S, A-G(O)		Have you ever/past year used a weapon, force, or strongarm methods to get money or things from someone?	No/yes	N/A
Aggravated assault (Y)	SRD	G-P(Y), A-F(M), S, A-G(O)		Have you ever/past year attacked someone with a weapon or with the intention of seriously hurting them?	No/yes	N/A
Violence (3) (PY)	CBCL, SRD	S, A-P(Y), S, A-F(M), S, A-G(O)		Caretaker: Gang fights Youth: In the past year have you been in a gang fight? Used a weapon, force, or strongarm methods to get money or things from someone? Attacked someone with a weapon or with the intention of seriously hurting them?	3-Point Likert No/yes	N/A
Burglary (Y)	SRD	S, A-P(Y), S, A-F(M), S, A-G(O)		Have you ever/past year gone into a building to steal something?	No/yes	N/A
Vehicle theft (Y)	SRD	G-P(Y), A-F(M), S, A-G(O)		Have you ever/past year stolen or tried to steal a motor vehicle?	No/yes	N/A
Theft from person (Y)	SRD	S, A-P(Y), S, A-F(M), S, A-G(O)		Have you ever/past year stolen a purse or picked a pocket?	No/yes	N/A

(continued)

Table 2.3 (continued)

Risk factor (respondent)[a] Source	Instrument[b]	Waves[c]	No. of items[d]	Example questions	Answer Scale or cutoff	Alpha (for scales)[d]
Theft from car (Y)	SRD	S, A-P(Y) S, A-F(M) S, A-G(O)		Have you ever/past year taken anything from a car that did not belong to you?	No/yes	N/A
Theft (4) (Y)	SRD	S, A-P(Y) S, A-F(M) S, A-G(O)		Have you ever/past year gone into a building to steal something? Stolen or tried to steal a motor vehicle? Taken anything from a car that did not belong to you?	No/yes	N/A
Shoplifting (PY)	SRD, CBCL	S, A-P(Y) S, A-F(M) S, A-G(O)		Parent: Shoplifts Youth: Have you ever/past year taken something from a store without paying?	No/yes 3-Point Likert	N/A
Other theft (Y)	SRD	S, A-P(Y) S, A-F(M) S, A-G(O)		Have you ever/past year stolen anything?	No/yes	NA
Receiving stolen property (Y)	SRD	G-P(Y) A-F(M) S, A-G(O)		Have you ever/past year knowingly bought, sold, or held stolen goods?	No/yes	N/A
Arson (PY)	SRD, CBCL	S, A-P(Y) S, A-F(M) S, A-G(O)		Youth: Have you ever/past year purposely set fire to a building or other property? Parent: Sets fires	No/yes 3-Point Likert	N/A
Vandalism (PTY)	SRD, CBCL	S, A-P(Y) S, A-F(M) S, A-G(O)		Youth: Have you ever/past year purposely damaged or destroyed property that did not belong to you? Parent, teacher: Vandalism	No/yes 3-Point Likert	N/A

Minor fraud (Y)	SRD	S, A-P(Y) S, A-F(M) S, A-G(O)	Have you ever/past year avoided paying for things such as movies, bus rides, food, or computer service? Tried to cheat someone by selling them something that was not what you said it was?	No/yes	N/A
Tobacco use (Y)	Drug consumption	S, A-P(Y) S, A-F(M) S, A-G(O)	Have you ever/in the past year smoked or chewed tobacco?	No/yes	N/A
Alcohol use (Y)	Drug consumption	S, A-P(Y) S, A-F(M) S, A-G(O)	Have you ever/in the past year drunk beer? wine? liquor?	No/yes	N/A
Marijuana use (Y)	Drug consumption	S, A-P(Y) S, A-F(M) S, A-G(O)	Have you ever/in the past year used marijuana?	No/yes	N/A
Hard drug use (Y)	Drug consumption	G-P(Y) A-F(M) S, A-G(O)	Have you ever/in the past year used tranquilizers without a prescription? Barbiturates? Codeine? Amphetamines? Any other prescription drugs? Crack cocaine? Other cocaine? Hallucinogens? Heroin? PCP?	No/yes	N/A
Drunk in public (Y)	SRD	G-P(Y) A-F(M) S, A-G(O)	In the past 6 months, have you been drunk in a public place?	No/yes	N/A
Drug (3) (Y)	SRD Drug consumption	G-P(Y) A-F(M) S, A-G(O)	Have you ever/in the past year sold marijuana or hashish? Sold hard drugs such as heroin, cocaine, or LSD? Used marijuana? Used hallucinogens? Used cocaine or crack? used heroin? Used PCP? Used tranquilizers, barbiturates, codeine, amphetamines, other prescription drugs without prescription?	No/yes	N/A
Arrests (official record)	Official records	Up to 2002	Official record of arrest for each category of offense	Count	

(continued)

Table 2.3 (continued)

Risk factor (respondent)[a] Source	Instrument[b]	Waves[c]	No. of items[d]	Example questions	Answer Scale or cutoff	Alpha (for scales)[d]
Convictions (official record)	Official records	up to 2002		Official record of conviction for each category of offense	Count	
Birth factors:						
Prenatal problems (P)	Birth Questionnaire	C	15	During pregnancy... high blood pressure? Infection associated with pregnancy? Take illicit drugs? How much weight did you gain?	No/yes	N/A
Mother's cigarette use during pregnancy (P)	Birth Questionnaire	C	1	Did you smoke cigarettes during pregnancy?	No/yes	N/A
Mother's alcohol use during pregnancy (P)	Birth Questionnaire	C	1	If you drank alcohol during pregnancy, how much did you drink (drinks per week):	>1 Drink/week	N/A
Family factors:						
Poor supervision (PY) Loeber, Farrington et al. (1998)	Supervision/ Involvement Scale	A	8	Parent: If you/another adult is not in home, does he leave note/call to let you know where he is going? Do you know whom he is with when he is not in home? Youth: If parent(s) not in home, do you leave note/call about where you are going? Do parent(s) know you are with when not in home?	3-Point Likert	0.56 (Y) 0.62 (M) 0.67 (O)
Poor communication (PY) – youngest cohort (P report only) Loeber, Farrington et al. (1998)	Revised Parent – Adolescent Communication Form	A	30 (Y) 49 (MO)	Parent: Get honest answers when you ask son questions? Very easy to express true feelings to him? Insults you when he is angry with you? Youth: You admit mistakes without trying to hide them from your father? Have your say when mother disagrees?	3-Point Likert	0.85 (Y) 0.86 (M) 0.90 (O)

Construct	Scale			Items	Response	Reliability
Physical punishment (PY) Loeber, Farrington et al. (1998)	Discipline Scale	A	3	Caretaker: If your son does something not allowed/ you do not like, do you slap, spank or hit him with something? Youth: If you do something you are not allowed/parents do not like, does mother slap, spank or hit you with something? …Does your father…?	3-Point Likert	N/A
Counter control (P) Loeber, Farrington et al. (1998)	Counter Control Scale	A	11	Behavior worsens after punishment? Worry that discipline makes him stubborn? Hesitate to discipline because you fear he will harm someone?	3-Point Likert	0.78 (Y) 0.78 (M) 0.81 (O)
Child abuse Stouthamer-Loeber et al. (2001b, 2002)	Allegheny County Children and Youth Services	Year 1994	1	Substantiated case of abuse on file when data collected in 1994, covering ages: Birth to age 12 youngest cohort Birth to age 16 middle cohort Birth to age 18 oldest cohort	No/yes	N/A
Boy not involved (PY) Loeber, Farrington et al. (1998)	Supervision/ Involvement Scale	A	8	Parent: Son helps plan family activities? Likes to get involved in family activities? Youth: You go to movies, sports, other events with family? Religious observances?	3-Point Likert	0.61 (Y) 0.62 (M) 0.73 (O)
Poor relationship with caretaker (PY) Loeber, Farrington et al. (1998)	Child's Relationship with Parent/ Siblings Scale	A	29	Parent: Felt you needed a vacation from your son? Wished you never had him? Got along with him? Youth: Thought mother really good? Wished father would leave you alone? Liked being your mother's kid?	3-Point Likert	0.86 (Y) 0.85 (M) 0.89 (O)
High parental stress (P) Cicchetti (1987, personal communication) and Loeber, Farrington et al. (1998)	Perceived Stress Scale	A	14	Successfully dealt with irritating life hassles? Felt things were going your way? Felt problems piling up?	3-Point Likert	0.82 (Y) 0.83 (M) 0.83 (O)

(continued)

Table 2.3 (continued)

Risk factor (respondent)[a] Source	Instrument[b]	Waves[c]	No. of items[d]	Example questions	Answer Scale or cutoff	Alpha (for scales)[d]
Parent substance use (P) Loeber, Farrington et al. (1998)	Family Health Questionnaire	A	1	Does mother or father (living in household or absent) have/ever had/ever sought help for alcohol or drug problems?	No/yes	N/A
Father behavior problems (P) Loeber, Farrington et al. (1998)	Family Health Questionnaire	A	1	Does father (living in household or absent) have/ever had/ever sought help for behavior problems?	No/yes	N/A
One or more relatives with police contact (P)	Family Criminal History	C	1	Siblings, biological and step/acting parents, aunts or uncles ever had contact with police (due to criminal behavior)?	No/yes	N/A
Peer factors:						
Bad friends (PY) Loeber, Farrington et al. (1998)	Parents and Peers Scale	A	10	Parent: Disapprove of son's friends? Friends a bad influence on him? Youth: Anything friends do that parents do not want you to do? Parents told you not to spend time with any of your friends?	No/yes	0.61 (Y) 0.72 (M) 0.75 (O)
Peer delinquency (Y) Loeber, Farrington et al. (1998)	Peer Delinquency Scale	A	9 (Y) 11 (MO)	In the past 6 months, how many of your friends... lied/disobeyed/talked back? Damaged property? Attacked someone with weapon?	3-Point Likert	0.82 (Y) 0.84 (M) 0.90 (O)
Peer substance use (Y) Loeber, Farrington et al. (1998)	Peer Delinquency Scale	H (Y) A (MO)	4	In the past 6 months, how many of your friends used... Alcohol? Marijuana? Hard Drugs? Sold hard drugs?	5-Point Likert	0.86 (Y) 0.52 (M) 0.68 (O)
Bad relationship with peers (PTY)	CBCL, TRF, YSR	S and A	3	Compared to others his age, how well does he get along with other children?	3-Point Likert	

School factors:

Construct	Instrument		#	Question	Scale	
Low academic achievement (PT) Achenbach and Edelbrock (1979, 1983) Edelbrock and Achenbach (1984) Achenbach and Edelbrock, (1987)	CBCL TRF YSR (oldest)	S and A	22	Parent: In past 6 months, how did your son do in… Reading or English? Writing? Teacher: Current school performance… Spelling? Math?	4-Point Likert	N/A
Low academic achievement (California Achievement Test)	California Achievement Test	S		Reading score, language score, math score	Percentile	N/A
Old for the grade (P) Loeber, Farrington et al. (1998)	Demographic Questionnaire	S	1	What is his date of birth? [He is "old" if >6 years old on September 1 in 1st grade, >9 in 4th grade, >12 in 7th grade.]	No/yes	N/A
Truancy (PYT) Loeber, Farrington et al. (1998)	CBCL, TRF, YSR, SRA/SRD	S and A	6	Parent and Teacher: Truancy, skips school Youth: Have you skipped classes or school without an excuse?	3-Point Likert No/yes	N/A
Suspended (PY)	CBCL, SRA/SRD	S and A	2	Parent: Suspended from school Youth: Ever/past year sent home from school for bad behavior?	3-Point Likert No/yes	N/A

Demographic factors:

Construct	Instrument		#	Question	Scale	
Broken family[c] (P) Loeber, Farrington et al. (1998)	Demographic Questionnaire	S and A	4	How are you related to the boy? How is your partner related to the boy?	Bio. or other	N/A
Low SES (P) Loeber, Farrington et al. (1998)	Demographic Questionnaire	A	6	Parent (for self and partner): Years of education? Highest degree? What is/was current/previous occupation?	Hollingshead definitions	N/A
Family on welfare (P) Loeber, Farrington et al. (1998)	Financial Information Questionnaire	A	1	Over the last year, has the household or anyone in the household received welfare?	No/yes	N/A
African American (P) Loeber, Farrington et al. (1998)	Demographic Questionnaire	S	1	What is the study child's race?	African American/ Caucasian	N/A
Young mother (P) Loeber, Farrington et al. (1998)	Demographic Questionnaire	G	1	How old were you when your first child was born?	Cutoff <20	N/A

(continued)

Table 2.3 (continued)

Risk factor (respondent)[a] / Source	Instrument[b]	Waves[c]	No. of items[d]	Example questions	Answer Scale or cutoff	Alpha (for scales)[d]
Bad neighborhood / US Bureau of Census	1990 US Census Tract Information	A	6	Median family income, % unemployed, % poverty, % ages 10–14, % single female-headed households with children, % divorced	Cutoff 25%	N/A
Bad neighborhood (P) / Loeber, Farrington et al. (1998)	Neighborhood Scale	A	17	Which are problems in your neighborhood: Unemployment? Racial conflict? Vandalism? Disrespect for authority?	3-Point Likert	0.95 (Y) 0.95 (M) 0.94 (O)
Large family (Y) / Loeber, Farrington et al. (1998)	Relationship with others	A	1	How many other children have lived with you during the past 6 months?	Number	N/A
Small house (P) / Loeber, Farrington et al. (1998)	Financial Information	A	1	How many rooms are in your home, including kitchen and bathrooms?	Cutoff <6	N/A
Unemployed mother (P) / Loeber, Farrington et al. (1998)	Demographic Questionnaire	A	1	In the past 6 months, how many weeks have you been unemployed?	Cutoff 25%	N/A

Notes:

[a] *P* parent, *T* teacher, *Y* youth

[b] *CBCL* Child Behavior Checklist (Achenbach & Edelbrock, 1979; Achenbach & Edelbrock 1983); *TRF* Teacher Report Form of the Child Behavior Checklist (Edelbrock & Achenbach, 1984); *YSR* Youth Self-Report (Achenbach & Edelbrock, 1987); *SRD* Self-Reported Delinquency Questionnaire (Elliott, Huizinga, & Ageton, 1985); *SRA* Self-Reported Antisocial Behavior Scale (Loeber, Stouthamer-Loeber, Van Kammen, & Farrington, 1989); Recent Mood and Feelings Questionnaire (Angold et al., 1996); *DISC-P* Diagnostic Interview Schedule for Children – Parent Version (Costello, Edelbrock, Kalas, Kessler, & Klaric, 1982; Costello, Edelbrock, & Costello, 1985); Child abuse/neglect collected from Allegheny County Children and Youth Services in 1994 and described in Stouthamer-Loeber, Loeber, Homish, and Wei (2001b) and Stouthamer-Loeber, Wei, Homish, and Loeber (2002). All other instruments described in: Loeber, Farrington et al. (1998)

[c] Ages of participants at waves 1 and 2 combined: youngest cohort = 7, middle cohort = 10, oldest cohort = 13. Ages at wave 4 = 8, youngest cohort; 11, middle cohort; 14, oldest cohort. Ages at wave 6 = 9, youngest cohort; 12, middle cohort; 15, oldest cohort
Cumulative data across waves 1–7 = ages 7–10 youngest cohort; ages 10–13 middle cohort; ages 13–16 oldest cohort. Cumulative data across waves 1–13 = ages 7–15 youngest cohort. Cumulative data across waves 9–13 = ages 11–15 youngest cohort. Child abuse data measured from birth until 1994 (youngest cohort, age 13; middle cohort, age 16; oldest cohort, age 19)

[d] *(Y)* youngest cohort, *(M)* middle cohort, *(O)* oldest cohort

[e] Formerly this construct was called "One or no biological parents in the home" (Loeber et al., 2008)

Chapter 3
Homicide Offenders and Victims in the USA, Pennsylvania, Pittsburgh, and the Pittsburgh Youth Study

Rolf Loeber, Erin Dalton, and David P. Farrington

Knowledge about homicide offenders and victims is dependent on the sources of information used and on the geographic location. This volume concerns homicide offenders and victims in the Pittsburgh Youth Study, a longitudinal study started in Pittsburgh, Pennsylvania (see Chap. 2) in 1987. Some critics may argue that this is a special, relatively small location and that characteristics of offenders and victims in the City of Pittsburgh may not apply to county, state, or national figures. Thus, the key questions for this chapter are:

- How common are homicides in Pittsburgh, and how do they compare regionally and nationally?
- How representative are homicide offenders in the PYS compared to homicide offenders in Allegheny County (where Pittsburgh is located), Pennsylvania, and the USA?
- What is the most common type of homicide offender in this study?
- What were the circumstances surrounding the homicide crimes, motives of offenders, and weapons used? (also addressed in Chap. 7)

To answer these questions, we present the characteristics of homicide offenders and victims in the Pittsburgh Youth Study (PYS) and homicide offenders elsewhere.[1] To illustrate real-life cases, we also present several case studies of homicide offenders and victims from the PYS. We primarily review data on homicide but also include some information on violence in general.

---

[1] Analyses of Pittsburgh and Allegheny County were carried out up to 2007 by the second author using data available at the Allegheny County Department of Health (see Dalton, Yonas, Warren, & Sturman, 2009).

R. Loeber and D.P. Farrington, *Young Homicide Offenders and Victims*,
Longitudinal Research in the Social and Behavioral Sciences: An Interdisciplinary Series,
DOI 10.1007/978-1-4419-9949-8_3, © Springer Science+Business Media, LLC 2011

Homicide Offenders and Victims

The USA. In the most recent overview of homicide in the USA (Fox & Zawitz, 2007), the national homicide victimization rate in 2005 was 5.6 homicides per 100,000 individuals, which translates to nearly 17,000 homicides for that year (16,692). This figure reflects annual homicide trends since 1998. Over the past 10 years, 167,614 individuals have been murdered in the USA. Knowledge of this incredible toll is not widespread, and remedial actions to reduce the numbers are intermittent at best (discussed more in detail in Chap. 10).

Homicide rates follow the age–crime curve and tend to increase during late adolescence, peak in early adulthood, and then decline (Farrington, 1986; Mercy, Rosenberg, Powell, Broome, & Roper, 1993). Many aspects of homicide have not substantially changed over the past decades in the USA (Fox & Zawitz, 2007): nearly all homicides are committed by males; most are perpetrated by African American male offenders against African American male victims; and, in most cases, the victim knew the offender. Although racial disparities in homicide are not fixed, they are pronounced. The homicide victimization rate for African Americans peaked at more than 37 per 100,000 between 1990 and 1993. It then gradually decreased to the low 20s and remained stable through 2005 at a rate of 20.6, which was over six times the rate for Caucasians (3.3). However, racial disparities are more pronounced for specific age groups. In 2005, the homicide rate for 14- to 17-year-old African American males was 26.4 (six times the rate for Caucasians of 4.4); for 18- to 24-year-old African American males, the rate jumped to 102.0, eight times higher (12.2) than the homicide rate for Caucasian males of the same age (Fox & Zawitz, 2007). This indicates that 1 in 1,000 young African American males is killed each year.

Guns are the most commonly used weapon in homicides (Fox & Zawitz, 2007; Snyder & Sickmund, 2006; Teplin, McClelland, Abram, & Mileusnic, 2005). Homicides by males are much more common between friends or acquaintances than between family members or between strangers, and most involve only one offender and one victim; homicides involving multiple offenders or victims are relatively rare.

Interpersonal arguments are the most commonly identified motivation for homicide. Felony homicides (i.e., homicide committed during the commission of another felony, such as robbery or burglary) are less common, as are gang-related homicides. However, guns are used more frequently in gang-related homicides than in felony- and argument-related homicides. Nationally, in 2005, 8,478 homicides were committed with a handgun and 2,868 with another type of gun; these figures have been fairly constant since 1998. Young homicide offenders are more likely to use a gun than another weapon or method (youth aged 14–18 used guns in 1,193 of the 1,611 homicides they committed in 2005; those aged 19–24 used guns in 5,790 out of 7,714 incidents). Thus, one in six of all gun-related homicides (17%) in the 14–24 age range of offenders were committed by individuals under age 18 who are not legally permitted to carry guns. Official figures regarding the number of homicides committed by known felons, who are also prohibited from carrying a gun, are unavailable.

Across the USA for the period 1976–2005, over half of the homicides occurred in cities with a population of 100,000 or more, whereas almost one quarter of the homicides took place in cities with a population of over one million (http://www.ojp.gov/bjs/homicide/city.htm, accessed March 24, 2009).

Pennsylvania, Allegheny County, and Pittsburgh. We examined the extent to which the national figures of homicide compare with homicide in Pennsylvania, Allegheny County, and Pittsburgh. Pennsylvania State Police data, collected according to the Uniform Crime Report standards, include information on incidents, victims, offenders, relationships, weapons, and motives, and were used primarily to provide information on offenders. These data are reliable between the years of 2000 and 2007.

In Pennsylvania, violence has steadily increased since the late 1990s; the state saw an 11% increase in homicides by firearms over the period of 1999–2004, and firearm injuries increased 5% between 1999 and 2003. Violence levels are highest in Allegheny County and Philadelphia County: Philadelphia County had 274 homicides by firearms in 2003 alone. Figures are lower in Pittsburgh, but remain second-highest in the state. The 5-year average homicide victimization rate for the period ending 2006 was 17 per 100,000 in Pittsburgh and 24 per 100,000 in Philadelphia.

Data regarding violence and homicide offending and victimization in Pennsylvania, Allegheny County, and Pittsburgh were gathered from a variety of regional sources. City of Pittsburgh Bureau of Police records from 1997 to 2007 provided information on all homicides and aggravated assaults with a firearm that were investigated by the City Police. Homicide data include the date, time, location of offense, census tract, and the victim's race, sex, and age. In 2003, the City of Pittsburgh Bureau of Police changed the way they characterized certain subsets of aggravated assaults (e.g., aggravated assault with an injury and drive-by shootings). Therefore, aggravated assault data predating 2003 cannot be accurately compared to more recent data.

Information was also extracted from the Allegheny County Medical Examiner's Office (ACME) data for the years 1997–2007 and the ACME Annual Reports for the years 2003 and 2006. The ACME is required to autopsy all premature and unexplained deaths that may have resulted from a sudden, violent, unexplained, or traumatic event. Incident information and victim demographics were manually compiled from the ACME records. It should be noted that the ACME data do not always agree with the City Police data but they add depth to this investigation by providing more information about the victims and the offenders, including information on homicides that occurred outside the City of Pittsburgh.

Violence Trends in Pittsburgh and Allegheny County. Scholars and politicians have paid much attention to the peaking of the US violent crime rate around 1993 and the subsequent national decline in homicides (e.g., Fox & Zawitz, 2007), but less discussed is the gradual increase in serious crime seen in several US cities in recent years. Pittsburgh has experienced the latter trend; homicides in the city peaked in 1993 and in Allegheny County they peaked 10 years later, in 2003. Between 1985 and 2007, the number of homicides in Pittsburgh has increased from an average of 40 per year to an average of over 60 per year (Fig. 3.1) in a population that was

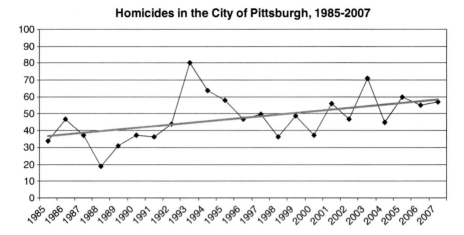

Fig. 3.1 Homicide trends in Pittsburgh, 1985–2007. *Source*: Dalton et al. (2009)

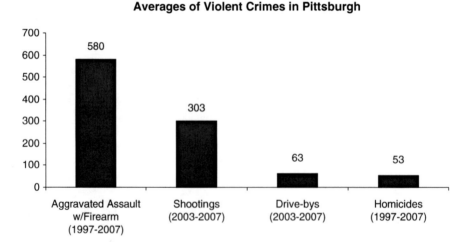

Fig. 3.2 Aggravated assault with a gun, shootings, drive-bys, and homicides (yearly averages). *Source*: Dalton et al. (2009)

decreasing during that period. In the 10 years up to 2007, an average of 55% of the homicides in Allegheny County occurred within the City of Pittsburgh, which makes up just 25% of Allegheny County's total population, demonstrating the dispropor-tionately urban nature of murders.

Although homicides represent an acute and highly visible indicator of commu-nity violence, more numerous indicators include aggravated assaults with a gun and aggravated assaults with a gun leading to injury. Figure 3.2 shows that, among these indicators, aggravated assault with a firearm was the most common, compared with shootings, while homicides were the rarest forms of violence.[2]

Who Are the Homicide Offenders and Victims in Pittsburgh?

Homicide Offenders. The age, race, and gender of homicide offenders in Pittsburgh was known in approximately half of all cases and these data suggest that offenders are demographically similar to victims: between 2000 and 2007, 51% of the suspects were under age 25, 80% were African American, and almost all (93%) were male. The majority of homicide offenders (88%) had a prior arrest or criminal record. The most recent data report that the average number of prior arrests per homicide offender was six; 64% had a prior drug arrest and 45% had a prior gun arrest (City of Pittsburgh Bureau of Police, 2002).

Relationships Between Homicide Offenders and Victims. Most of the homicides between 2000 and 2007, where the race of both the offender and victim was known (51% of cases), involved an offender and victim of the same race: 74% of these were perpetrated by an African American offender against an African American victim and 11% involved a Caucasian offender and a Caucasian victim. Interracial incidents were far less common: 7% of homicides involved a Caucasian offender and an African American victim, and 6% involved an African American offender and a Caucasian victim.

Offenders and victims were also most likely to be of the same gender: for homicide cases in which the gender of both parties was known (32% of cases), the majority involved a male offender and a male victim (77%). In contrast, homicides involving a male offender and a female victim were less common (16%). In the rare incidents involving a female offender, male victims were more common than female victims (5% vs. 2%).

In cases where the relationship between the victim and the offender was recorded (32% of cases), victims usually knew their killer in some way. In 79% of incidents, the victim and offender were acquaintances (45%), family (16%), or friends/neighbors (18%); only 21% of homicides occurred between strangers.

Characteristics of the Homicides. Between 2000 and 2007, 80% of homicides in Pittsburgh were committed with a firearm, and more than one-third of those were committed with an automatic weapon (36%). About one in ten homicides (9%) were committed with a knife, and the remainder involved the use of a blunt object, fire, strangulation, or other method of killing.

Homicides were most often committed between a single offender and a single victim. Incidents involving multiple victims or multiple offenders were extremely rare (1 and 5 out of 471, respectively). Shootings and homicides during the period

---

[2] Note that the numbers in Fig. 3.2 are not fully comparable because of different observation periods.

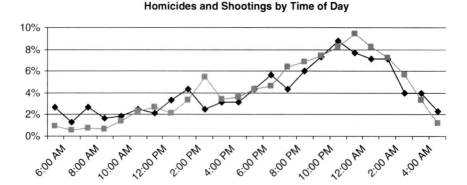

Fig. 3.3 Homicides and shootings by time of day in Pittsburgh. *Source*: Dalton et al. (2009). Note: Homicides (1997–2007); Shootings (2003–2007)

2003–2007 were slightly more common during the summer months (June, July, and August) than during the rest of the year. On an average day, the frequency of shootings increased almost linearly from 10:00 a.m. onward, then peaked at midnight and linearly decreased until 5:00 a.m. (see Fig. 3.3).

Location of Violence. Homicides tend to cluster in the most disadvantaged neighborhoods. In Allegheny County, the highest homicide concentrations were found in the municipalities bordering the City of Pittsburgh or within deprived City neighborhoods.

Table 3.1 presents the number of homicides and the homicide rate per 100,000 persons for each of Allegheny County's municipalities outside the City of Pittsburgh for the years 1997–2007 (based on the location of the incident). Wilkinsburg had the highest homicide rate (69 per 100,000), followed by Braddock (28) and Duquesne (23). Seven other municipalities had murder rates between 13 and 19 per 100,000, further illustrating the enormous geographic concentration of homicides in Allegheny County. The municipalities with the highest homicide rates are also the municipalities with the highest concentration of African American residents; Wilkinsburg and Braddock each have 67% African American residents, while Duquesne has 48%.

Homicides are similarly clustered in a few neighborhoods within the City of Pittsburgh. Table 3.2 summarizes the distribution of homicide victimization throughout Pittsburgh neighborhoods and ranks those communities by the highest number of homicides and the highest rate of homicides per 100,000 residents (based on the location of the incident). The neighborhoods of Homewood, the Hill District, and the North Side experienced the highest levels of victimization. Of the killings committed within the City of Pittsburgh, Homewood (Homewood South, Homewood

Table 3.1 Homicides and homicide rates in municipalities outside of the City of Pittsburgh

Municipality	Number of homicides (1997–2007)	Municipality	Homicide rate (per 100,000)
Wilkinsburg	51	Wilkinsburg	69
Penn Hills	31	Braddock	28
McKeesport	26	Duquesne	23
Duquesne	17	Wilmerding	19
Swissvale	11	Homestead	17
Clairton	10	Sharpsburg	17
North Braddock	9	East Pittsburgh	15
Monroeville	8	North Braddock	14
West Mifflin	8	Rankin	14
Braddock	8	Clairton	13
Carnegie	7	McKeesport	11
Sharpsburg	6	Carnegie	8

Table 3.2 Homicides and homicide rates in Pittsburgh neighborhoods, 1997–2007

Neighborhood	Number of Homicides	Neighborhood	Homicide rate (per 100,000)
Homewood South	41	South Shore	179
Middle Hill	24	Strip District	113
Larimer	21	Homewood South	112
East Hills	20	Middle Hill	112
Perry South	20	Homewood West	108
Hazelwood	19	Larimer	81
East Liberty	19	Terrace Village	61
Lincoln-Lemington Belmar	18	Crawford-Roberts	51
Garfield	17	California-Kirkbride	51
Terrace Village	16	East Hills	50
Crawford-Roberts	16	Beltzhoover	50

West, and Homewood North) accounted for 14% of total homicide victims, the Hill District (Middle Hill, Terrace Village, and Crawford-Roberts) for 11%, and the North Side (Perry South and Central Northside) for 6%.

The homicide rates in some Pittsburgh neighborhoods (e.g., South Shore, Strip District, Homewood South, Middle Hill, Homewood West, and Larimer) are even higher than in the municipalities described above; Homewood South had a homicide rate of 112 per 100,000 and eight other neighborhoods with substantial populations had homicide rates exceeding 50 per 100,000 persons (Table 3.2). Eight out of the nine neighborhoods with large populations are predominantly inhabited by African American individuals (78% or more). It is important to note that the extremely high homicide rates in the South Shore and the Strip District may be misleading, because these neighborhoods have small populations and many of the homicide victims did not live in these neighborhoods.

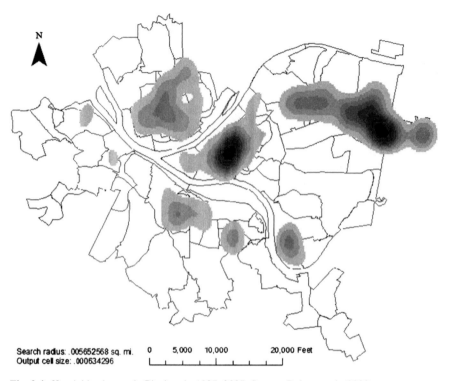

Search radius: .005652568 sq. mi.   0   5,000   10,000   20,000 Feet
Output cell size: .000634296

Fig. 3.4 Homicide clusters in Pittsburgh, 1997–2007. *Source*: Dalton et al. (2009)

Homicides tend to cluster even within the most violence-prone neighborhoods in the City of Pittsburgh. Geographic mapping and cluster analysis were used to identify patterns of violence in Allegheny County and Pittsburgh from 1997 to 2007. Geographic information on the location of each incident was used to create a geographic information system (GIS) to analyze the distribution of crime across Allegheny County municipalities and Pittsburgh neighborhoods, and map concentrations of crime. Figure 3.4 clearly demonstrates clusters of homicides within the highest homicide neighborhoods, such as Perry South on the North Side, Middle Hill and Terrace Village in the Hill District, and a large cluster in the adjoining Larimer, Homewood West, Homewood North, and Homewood South neighborhoods situated on the east side of the City. Two smaller clusters are visible in the Beltzhoover and Hazelwood neighborhoods, both on the South Side.

Figure 3.5 shows the shooting clusters in the City for the same period. Not surprisingly, the shooting clusters appear more frequently, but in the same neighborhoods, as the homicide clusters. A cluster map of aggravated assaults with a firearm for the same period, not shown here, demonstrates that these clusters also coincide with the shooting and homicide clusters. In other words, aggravated assaults, shootings,

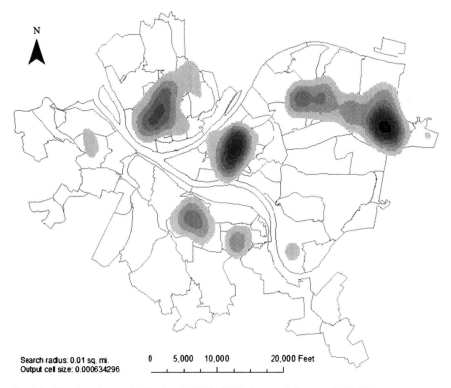

N

Search radius: 0.01 sq. mi.
Output cell size: 0.000634296

0   5,000   10,000   20,000 Feet

Fig. 3.5 Shooting clusters in Pittsburgh, 2003–2007. *Source*: Dalton et al. (2009)

and homicides during a 5-year period have been concentrated within certain neighborhoods, and even within certain areas of those neighborhoods.

Offenders' motivation to commit homicide is often difficult to define. The State Police data contain notes about motive(s) in only 43% of homicide cases over the period 2000–2006. The most commonly cited motives were arguments (50%) and burglary, robbery, and theft (20%). Other motives identified, albeit infrequently, include a felon killed by police or a citizen, narcotics, arson, sniper attack, and gang-related homicide. These data are not especially illuminating because the defined categories are so broad as to be uninformative (e.g., "argument" is not divided into types of or reasons for arguments). Further, the fact that gang-related motives are cited as often as sniper attacks suggests that more work is needed to accurately determine why violence occurs.

In summary, violence is a serious problem in the Pittsburgh region and disproportionately affects young African American men. Both homicide victims and offenders tend to live in a few disadvantaged neighborhoods and tend to have criminal backgrounds themselves. Guns are a major part of the problem; more than 80% of homicides are committed with firearms, and for every homicide there are about four shootings, many of which result in injury. Further studies are needed to understand why violence occurs, as motives are difficult to discern accurately from the police data.

Who Are the Victims of Homicide in Pittsburgh?

Between 1997 and 2007, about half of all homicide victims in the City of Pittsburgh were under age 25 and nearly all were African American (86%) and male (85%). Homicide victimization has increased for African Americans during this period, a trend not mirrored by a higher victimization rate for Caucasians. In 1997, the homicide rate for African Americans in the City of Pittsburgh was 39.6 per 100,000; by 2007, that rate had increased 153% to 60.6. The homicide rate for African Americans is alarmingly high, particularly considering that the demographic makeup of the City of Pittsburgh is 26% African American and 72% Caucasian; this shows that African Americans are significantly overrepresented in homicide victimization. The vulnerability of African American men is particularly troubling. In 2005, the US homicide rate was 5.6 per 100,000 (Fox & Zawitz, 2007), but it was 284.2 per 100,000 for young African American men living in Pittsburgh – 50 times the national average. Figure 3.6 demonstrates the disparity in homicide rates based on race, gender, and age. While African American men have the highest homicide rate across all age groups, they are most at risk between the ages of 16 and 36.

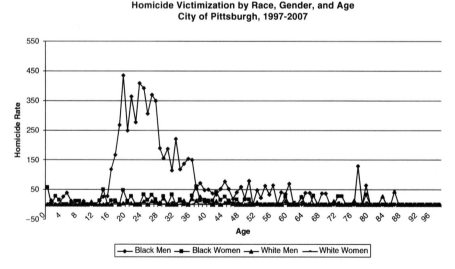

Fig. 3.6 Rate of homicide victimization by gender, race, and age per 100,000 people in Pittsburgh, 1997–2007. *Source*: Dalton et al. (2009)

Between 2003 and 2005, more than half of the homicide victims in Pittsburgh had criminal records themselves; 56% had criminal cases in the fifth judicial district.[3] Young adults (aged 25–34) were even more likely to have criminal records; 72% of 25- to 34-year-old victims and 70% of 35- to 44-year-old victims had engaged in some prior criminal activity.

There were distinct temporal patterns during the day in victimization based on specific age groups: for 13- to 17-year-olds, victimization peaked during the after-school hours, whereas for 18- to 24-year-olds, homicides were more common in the evenings and the late-night hours. Slightly more shootings took place on Sundays compared to other days of the week, but this too varied with the age of the victim. Those aged 17 and under were more likely to be killed on a weekday evening than at other times, whereas 18- to 24-year-old victims were more susceptible during the late-night hours throughout the week and on the weekend. For the most part, these trends follow the routine activity patterns of these age groups.

Many homicide victims live in economically depressed, high-crime neighborhoods, and municipalities. Data from the Allegheny County Medical Examiner's office for the period 1997–2007 show that 255, or 30%, of the 878 homicide victims resided in just 12 communities, many of which are categorized as severely distressed according to criteria developed by the Annie E. Casey Foundation.[4]

Homicide Offenders and Victims in the Pittsburgh Youth Study

Do the experiences of PYS participants reflect violence trends in Pittsburgh, Allegheny County, Pennsylvania, and the USA? Information about homicide offenders and victims in the PYS was obtained from searches of local, state, and federal criminal records, interviews with PYS participants and their families, searches of local newspapers, searches of the national Lexis-Nexis media database, and the local coroner's office.

Based on information collected up to May 30, 2009, 37 PYS males were convicted for homicide committed between ages 15 and 29. Table 3.3 shows the ages at which these homicides were committed (for the 36 convicted offenders who were known). The peak ages were at 18 (8 offenders) and 19 (11 offenders). The mean

---

[3] This implies that the analysis does not include offenses that might have occurred in the East of Pennsylvania or in another state.

[4] The Annie E. Casey Foundation describes severely distressed neighborhoods as those that have at least three of four high-risk criteria: high poverty, high percentage of female-headed families, high percentage of high school dropouts, and high percentage of working-age males unattached to the workforce. These criteria were used to determine the degree to which a homicide victim's neighborhood of residence was distressed; 27 communities within Allegheny County warranted this designation.

Table 3.3 Ages of homicide offenders and victims

Age	No. at risk	Convicted		Arrested		Victims	
		No.	Cum %	No.	Cum %	No.	Cum %
15	1,512	1	2.8	0	0.0	0	0.0
16	1,512	2	8.3	2	8.7	2	5.1
17	1,510	4	19.4	1	13.0	0	5.1
18	1,510	8	41.7	1	17.4	5	17.9
19	1,505	11	72.2	3	30.4	3	25.6
20	1,500	3	80.6	2	39.1	3	33.3
21	1,494	3	88.9	0	39.1	8	53.8
22	1,485	0	88.9	3	52.2	1	56.4
23	1,483	0	88.9	5	73.9	3	64.1
24	1,479	2	94.4	4	91.3	2	69.2
25	1,475	1	97.2	0	91.3	2	74.4
26	1,473	1	100.0	1	95.7	5	87.2
27	1,463	0	100.0	1	100.0	2	92.3
28	1,280	0	100.0	0	100.0	2	97.4
29	1,061	0	100.0	0	100.0	1	100.0
No.		36		23		39	
Mean age	31.6	19.7		22.0		22.7	

Note: No. at risk takes account of deaths and ages at May 30, 2009
Cum % = Cumulative %

age of offending was 19.7. Four-fifths of offenders had committed their homicides by age 20.

Table 3.3 also shows the number of males at risk at each age. Of the 1,517 males in the PYS, four died and one emigrated permanently by age 14. These males are considered to be not at risk of offending, leaving 1,512 males at risk at age 15. The number of males at risk then decreased because of deaths (57 males died up to age 29) and because not all males in the youngest cohort had reached their 30th birthday. On May 30, 2009, the mean age of the youngest cohort was 28.4, compared with 31.7 for the middle cohort, and 34.8 for the oldest cohort. Table 3.3 shows that almost all of the males were at risk of conviction up to age 27, but not all were at risk at ages 28 and 29. Therefore, one or two further convictions of males in the youngest cohort may yet occur.

Table 3.4 shows the years in which homicides were committed, from 1992 (the first homicide) to 2006 (the last). The average year was 1997. Three-quarters of the homicides were committed up to 1998. For comparability, national figures for arrests of persons aged 15–29 are also shown. These were kindly supplied by Matt Durose (2010) of the US Bureau of Justice Statistics. It can be seen that the number of young homicide arrestees decreased from the peak of 16,402 in 1993 to 8,665 in 2000, and since then has fluctuated to the figure of 8,574 in 2008.

The homicide conviction rate in a population does not fully represent the actual homicide rate due to several factors, including local case clearance and successful prosecution of suspected homicide offenders. Police must first identify potential

Table 3.4 Years of homicide offenders and victims

Year	Convicted		Arrested		Victims		USA	
	No.	Cum %	No.	Cum %	No.	Cum %	No. victims	No. arrested
1992	2	5.6	1	4.3	0	0.0	11,221	15,464
1993	5	19.4	2	13.0	4	10.3	11,648	16,402
1994	3	27.8	1	17.4	4	20.5	11,126	15,364
1995	6	44.4	1	21.7	4	30.8	10,087	14,728
1996	5	58.3	1	26.1	3	38.5	9,004	12,992
1997	5	72.2	2	34.8	4	48.7	8,412	12,683
1998	1	75.0	2	43.5	3	56.4	7,782	11,868
1999	3	83.3	5	65.2	2	61.5	7,028	9,801
2000	1	86.1	1	69.6	1	64.1	6,985	8,665
2001	3	94.4	4	87.0	4	74.4	7,362	8,924
2002	0	94.4	1	91.3	0	74.4	7,415	9,315
2003	1	97.2	1	95.7	2	79.5	7,684	8,534
2004	0	97.2	1	100.0	3	87.2	7,360	8,649
2005	0	97.2	0	100.0	0	87.2	7,760	9,224
2006	1	100.0	0	100.0	0	87.2	8,044	8,862
2007	0	100.0	0	100.0	1	89.7	7,858	9,010
2008	0	100.0	0	100.0	4[a]	100.0	7,305	8,574
No.	36		23		39			
Mean year	1997.0		1998.8		1999.4			

Notes: Mean year +0.5 to correct for integer years
No. of victims of homicide in USA aged 15–29
No. of arrested homicide offenders in USA aged 15–29 (both corrected for % of police agencies reporting each year) (*Source*: Durose, 2010, personal communication)
Cum % = Cumulative %
[a]Including one in January 2009

homicide offenders; these individuals then need to be tried in court by the district attorney's office. Farrington, Langan, and Tonry (2004) found that 84% of homicide offenders in cases recorded by the police were arrested (in 1996), while 66% of arrested homicide offenders were convicted of homicide.

Accurately calculating the PYS homicide rate requires a positive confirmation of both identity and conviction status. Since the conviction rate described above does not necessarily include all actual homicide offenders, the PYS rate is undoubtedly conservative. Further, we identified a group of 33 males who were arrested and charged with homicide by the police but who were not convicted of homicide. Some of these individuals may possibly be convicted in the future, but most were not convicted because they terrorized potential witnesses, because the evidence was too weak to secure a conviction in court, or because they were innocent. This group undoubtedly contains some actual homicide offenders. Thus, in addition to the convicted homicide offenders, we will pay some attention to those individuals who were arrested for homicide but not convicted.

Table 3.3 shows that the arrested homicide offenders committed their alleged offenses at an average age of 22 (where this was known). Three-quarters of their offenses were committed by age 23. Table 3.4 shows that the average year in which they committed their offenses was 1998. About 70% of their crimes were committed by 2000.

In total, 39 PYS males were victims of homicide. Table 3.3 shows that the most common age to be killed was 21, and the average age on death was 22.7. About 70% of these males were killed by age 24. Table 3.4 shows that the average year of death was 1999, and three-quarters of these males were killed by 2001. For comparability, Table 3.4 also shows national figures for victims of homicide aged 15–29. It can be seen that the number of young homicide victims decreased from the peak of 11,648 in 1993 to 6,985 in 2000, and since then has fluctuated to 7,305 in 2008.

Excluding five boys who were not at risk, the prevalence of convicted homicide offenders was 2.4% (37 out of 1,512), compared with 2.2% for arrestees, and 2.6% for victims. Weighting back to the Pittsburgh public school population, these prevalences became 2.0% for convicted offenders, 2.0% for arrested offenders, and 2.2% for homicide victims.

As expected from prior research (e.g., Cook & Laub, 1998; Fox & Zawitz, 2007), African American males were more involved in homicides than were Caucasian males. Of the 37 convicted homicide offenders, 32 were African American, compared with 31 of the 33 arrested offenders, and 37 of the 39 homicide victims. The prevalences of convicted homicide offenders were 3.7% of African American boys vs. 0.8% of Caucasian boys (weighted figures 3.2% vs. 0.5%). For arrested homicide offenders, the prevalences were 3.6% vs. 0.3% (weighted figures 3.3% vs. 0.3%). For homicide victims, the prevalences were 4.3% vs. 0.3% (weighted figures 3.7% vs. 0.3%). Unweighted data are used in this book, as the main interest is in studying predictions for individuals rather than making population estimates.

Focusing on weighted data for males aged 18–24, there were 21 African American and 3 Caucasian convicted homicide offenders, giving an annual homicide offending rate of 353 per 100,000 for African Americans and 65 per 100,000 for Caucasians (African American to Caucasian ratio 5.4). In the same age range, there were 18 African American and 2 Caucasian homicide victims, giving an annual homicide victimization rate of 303 per 100,000 for African American and 43 per 100,000 for Caucasians (African American to Caucasian ratio 7.0). Of course, all these figures would have large confidence intervals around them. These estimates of 300–350 homicide offenders and victims per 100,000 population are comparable to the rates for young African American males in Pittsburgh shown in Fig. 3.6.

This book focuses on 37 convicted homicide offenders, 33 arrested homicide offenders, and 39 homicide victims. Two convicted offenders and one arrested offender were also homicide victims. These groups are compared with 1,406 controls, excluding the five males who died or emigrated permanently by age 14.

The numbers of convicted homicide offenders were similar in the three age cohorts: 11 in the youngest, 13 in the middle, and 13 in the oldest cohort. However, there were fewer arrested homicide offenders in the youngest cohort (6), compared with 13 in the middle cohort, and 14 in the oldest cohort. Also, there were fewer homicide victims in the youngest cohort (9), compared with 13 in the middle cohort, and 17 in the oldest cohort.

It seems likely that there were fewer homicide offenders and victims in the youngest cohort because they went through their peak ages for homicide (16–24) during the years when the US homicide rate was decreasing (1996–2004), whereas the oldest cohort went through these ages during years when the US homicide rate was very high (1990–1998). It is possible that the number of convicted homicide offenders was not fewer in the youngest cohort because the police and courts in the City of Pittsburgh became more successful over time in securing convictions. The number of (arrested plus convicted) homicide offenders was lowest in the youngest cohort (17), compared with 26 in the middle cohort, and 27 in the oldest cohort.

Convicted Homicide Offenders

Information about the convicted homicide offenders and their offenses and victims was obtained from the sources listed above, namely criminal records, interviews, and the mass media. Information was not available for every offender about every topic. Chapter 7 provides additional information from interviews with the offenders.

Guns were used in the majority of homicide cases involving PYS participants (27). Other cases involved knife attacks (2), vehicular homicide (1), strangulation by a cord (1), arson (1), and beatings by hand (2), a brick (1), or a metal rod (1). The motives identified were retaliation (13), robbery (7), a drug deal gone wrong (5), a gang-related dispute (3), a domestic dispute (1), arson (1), and mental illness (1). Two-thirds of the offenders had some form of prior contact with the victim (22 out of 33 known).

Sixteen of the homicides were committed by a perpetrator acting alone, while 8 were committed by two offenders, and 11 were committed by three or more offenders. These figures for multiple-perpetrator homicides are much higher than the figures for Pittsburgh cited earlier in this chapter. There was only one victim in all cases except one, where three people were killed in an arson attack.

Six homicide offenders were convicted of first-degree murder, 6 of second-degree murder, and 17 of third-degree murder. There were three convictions for manslaughter, one for conspiracy to commit homicide, one for vehicular homicide, and one for a homicide of unknown degree. Sentence length varied: 12 offenders were sentenced to life imprisonment, and 3 of these were sentenced to life without parole. Of the remaining homicide offenders, 13 were sentenced to more than 10 years,[5] and 5 of these to more than 20 years.[6] Five offenders received sentences of less than 5 years. Two offenders did not receive a sentence because they were killed by others.

In agreement with prior research (e.g., Snyder & Sickmund, 1999), the overwhelming majority of the victims of PYS offenders were male (34 out of 36), and most were African American (21 out of 29 known). Cross-racial offenses were rare (7).

---

[5] This is based on the minimum of the range of the sentence (e.g., a sentence of 13–27 years).

[6] Also based on the minimum sentence.

Most homicide offenses involved African American males who killed other African American males (19 out of 29 known, or 56%). More than one-third of the victims (13 out of 38 known) were youths between the ages of 15 and 21, while another 9 were aged 22–29, and 14 were aged 30 or over. Two victims were aged 1 and 3.

Most convicted homicide offenders appeared fairly homogeneous. The offenses often involved guns, gangs, drugs, and African American males. However, four of the offenders seemed unusual. One was mentally ill, one committed arson, one committed a domestic homicide, and one committed a vehicular homicide. We considered excluding these four cases in the predictions but decided not to, in the interests of studying a representative sample of homicide offenders. Explorations showed that deleting these four cases did marginally improve some prediction exercises, no doubt because the homicide offenders became marginally more homogeneous.

Selected Case Histories of Convicted Homicide Offenders. Although this volume attempts to quantify risk factors for homicide offending and victimization, we are also interested in the kinds of people who commit murder and those who become victims. We therefore present some selected case histories here. To ensure confidentiality, we modified some aspects of the case histories; names and some other identifying details have been changed. The case histories focus on those types of homicides that were most common (i.e., relating to drugs, gangs, robbery, and retaliation) and exclude cases that were highly unusual (e.g., fire-fighters perishing after one participant set a house on fire to claim insurance money; a young man killing his girlfriend in a domestic violence dispute; and a young man killing a 3-year-old child).

Case 1: Robbery and Homicide. Sean was 18 when he and some friends robbed the victim, shooting him to avoid being identified later as the robbers. Sean had been born to a single, drug-using mother and came from a family of five, but he did not have contact with his biological father. At age 6, because of the bad situation in the home, Sean and the other children were placed in foster care. Sean had shown problematic behaviors from at least age 7 onward, including frequent lying, shoplifting, fighting, and disobedience at home and in school before age 11. He committed his first act of serious delinquency, breaking and entering, at age 11 and again at age 12, when he was first arrested. He was placed in a detention home at the age of 12, then again at 15 and 18. Sean did poorly in school and could not read at age 14. A psychiatric diagnosis at age 13 specified conduct disorder and learning disability. He had repeated run-ins with the law for a variety of delinquent acts, including drug possession, before being arrested for homicide at age 18.

Case 2: Gang-Related Homicide. Thomas was 15 years old when he and a few fellow gang members searched their neighborhood for members of a rival gang, then fired the shots that killed a 25-year-old man. Thomas's mother had married late and held clerical jobs, but was thought to drink excessively and use drugs. His biological father was incarcerated several times and had drug problems. Thomas's performance at school initially was poor but improved with time, but he displayed behavior problems (disobedience, fighting, and hot temper), leading to several suspensions. His mother did not approve of his friends, many of whom engaged in delinquent acts.

The family lived in a neighborhood that was severely disadvantaged and had a high crime rate. When he was a preschooler, Thomas displayed strong stubborn behavior, hyperactivity, disobedience, vandalism, and fighting with and bullying of peers. He was aged 11 when he first broke into a building. He carried a gun and had joined a gang by the time of the homicide.

Case 3: Retaliation and Homicide. Chuck and four of his fellow gang members attended the funeral of a friend who had been killed by an individual known to them. In retaliation, he shot a boy who apparently did not have anything to do with the killing. Chuck came from a two-parent family and both his parents had jobs. At home, Chuck showed persistent oppositional and conduct problems, was thought to be hyperactive, and started carrying a weapon at age 10. In school, Chuck showed behavior problems, including explosive and unpredictable behavior. His parents did not approve of his friends, but were unable to influence Chuck's associations with peers. He was first picked up by the police at age 11. Two years later, he became a gang member and took on a leadership role. He was 16 years old when he committed murder.

Case 4: Drug Dealing and Homicide. At age 21, Peter got into an argument with a drug dealer about drugs, and then shot the dealer. Peter came from a single-parent home. His mother had a string of male partners, one of whom abused her. She also had several other children by different men and was reported to be using drugs. Peter showed a range of oppositional and conduct problems as a child. Because of his mother's problems, he was removed from the family home at age 8 and was reared in several foster homes. He did well in school, but was repeatedly suspended because of misbehavior, and did not receive a diploma. Subsequently, he did not have a job and hung out with friends in a disadvantaged neighborhood. He was 11 years old when he first robbed someone, and 15 years old when he first burglarized a house. He was heavily involved in a variety of delinquent acts and started using alcohol and drugs before age 13.

Homicide Victims

Most of the information about homicide victims came from the local coroner's office, which provided detailed information about 32 of the 39 cases. The number of offenders was 1 in 20 cases, 2 in 2 cases, and 3 in 4 cases, totaling 36 offenders known. In 32 of these cases, the offender was known to have been charged with criminal homicide. The number of victims was 1 in 31 cases and 2 in 4 cases. All known offenders (36) were male. The race of the offender was recorded as African American in 29 cases and Caucasian in 5 cases. The age of the offender was 15–21 in 16 cases and 22–30 in 16 cases.

Almost all victims (36 out of 39) were killed by shooting, with two stabbings and one beating. According to the coroner's office, there was prior contact between victims and offenders in all cases except one. The victim was recorded as having alcohol in his blood in 13 out of 30 cases known, having drugs in 7 out of 20 cases, and having a weapon in 4 out of 24 cases. In general, the homicide victims seem quite homogeneous; 37 out of 39 were African American, and most cases involved drugs or guns or drinking or gangs or arguments or retaliation or robbery (and usually several of these). These types of homicides have often been identified in the literature (see, e.g., Cornell, Benedek, & Benedek, 1987; Roberts, Zgoba, & Shahidullah, 2007).

There were sometimes connections between victims and offenders. In two cases, one PYS male killed another PYS male. In another case, one PYS male was involved in a shootout in which another PYS male was killed. In two cases, two PYS males were killed together. In another case, two PYS males were shot in a drive-by shooting and one died. In another case, two PYS males and a man (A) shot another man, and then (A) was killed by another PYS male. In yet another case, one PYS male and a man (B) killed a 15-year-old boy, and then (B) killed another PYS male. Finally, one PYS male and a man (C) killed someone, and then (C) together with another PYS male shot and paralyzed a boy.

Selected Case Histories of Homicide Victims. The following case histories pertain to victims of homicide who had been participants in the PYS. As before, to preserve confidentiality, names and some details have been changed.

Case History 1: Victimization and Robbery. At the age of 23, John was shot and killed during an armed robbery. He and two friends were approached on the street by an unknown assailant and ordered to lie on the ground in a prone position. Robbing John and his friends of money and personal items, the assailant shot John in the head. Although none of the victims resisted in any way, John was the only person who was shot. This led the police to believe that this incident had not been a random act of violence and was likely retaliation against the victim. At the time of his death, John was being sought on warrants for multiple felony narcotic violations.

Case History 2: Victimization and Arrest History. Carl was shot at point-blank range outside a garage. He had a lengthy arrest history dating back to his early childhood years; he had been arrested 12 times by the age of 14. The majority of his arrests were for possession or sales of drugs. However, he also had been arrested for theft, auto theft, disorderly conduct, and aggravated assault. Early in life, he lived with his mother, but the whereabouts of his father were not known. He completed high school and 2 years of college, but quit and became unemployed. At the time of his death at age 21, he had three children by his girlfriend.

Case History 3: Victimization and Nonoffending. Bill was killed in an execution type of killing at age 23. He had a minimal delinquent record, but had reported that half of his friends used marijuana and engaged in delinquent acts. He was brought up by a single mother, and completed high school. At the time of his death, he was employed full-time as a store supervisor. At that time, he was married and had a son and a daughter.

Case History 4: Victimization and Revenge. Jeffrey was killed by a man who was looking for Jeffrey's uncle, and shot him instead, apparently in revenge for an alleged killing by his uncle. Jeffrey had a lengthy criminal history since age 14, which brought him repeatedly into contact with the police and the court, even as an adult. He left school early but, at the time of his death at age 21, he was working full time as a waiter in a restaurant. He lived with his mother and had very few friends who engaged in delinquent acts.

Conclusions

We reviewed homicide offending and victimization in the PYS against the backdrop of violence and homicide in Pittsburgh, Allegheny County, Pennsylvania, and the USA. The homicide rate peaked in Pittsburgh in 1993, then decreased, but since then has gradually increased over the next 14 years. It is in this time window that the majority of the murders by participants in the PYS have been committed. It is also the time window in which participants of the PYS became victims of homicide.

The findings reported in this chapter indicate that homicide offenders and homicide victims in the PYS closely resemble homicide offenders and victims in Allegheny County in which Pittsburgh is situated. The major points of resemblance are: almost all of the homicide offenders and homicide victims tend to be male with an overrepresentation of African American males. The majority in each group is known to the police and the court, and tends to have a criminal record. The majority of the homicides are African American males killing African American males, and the majority of the killings are by means of a firearm. The killings were clustered in the most disadvantaged neighborhoods. Where known, the motives for the homicides usually involved gangs, guns, drugs, alcohol, arguments, retaliation, and/or robbery. The predominant characteristic of the homicides committed by and against PYS participants might be characterized as "street homicides."

Where possible, we also compared the extent to which murders in the PYS resembled those reported nationally in the USA. Again, the comparisons are very similar, and support the notion that the homicide offenders and victims in the PYS constitute a microcosm of what happens elsewhere. At the same time, we should emphasize that the comparisons between the PYS homicide offenders and victims and those in other locations have limitations, especially because of the modest numbers of homicide offenders and victims in the PYS.

On the positive side, however, questions investigated in the following chapters are key issues that apply to young homicide offenders and victims in any location in the USA, especially in large metropolitan areas of which Pittsburgh is one. Most importantly, unlike other data sets on homicide offenders and victims, the PYS offers unique information about the early risk factors and problem behaviors of homicide offenders and victims, the ways they were reared, their educational achievements, and many other aspects of their lives prior to the homicide event. The value of examining homicide offenders and victims in the PYS is all the greater because of the relatively high rate of homicide offenders and victims in the sample, especially among the African American males.

Chapter 4
Early Risk Factors for Convicted Homicide Offenders and Homicide Arrestees

David P. Farrington and Rolf Loeber

As mentioned in Chap. 1, research on the prediction of convicted homicide offenders using prospective data is extraordinarily rare. In 2005, we published the first paper on the prospective prediction of convicted homicide offenders in a population sample (Loeber et al., 2005a). The analyses in this chapter differ from that paper in several major ways. First, the 2005 paper had a smaller number of homicide offenders, with four new cases having become evident since then. Second, the 2005 paper analyzed weighted data, reducing the number of convicted homicide offenders to only 23. Third, the prediction exercise in the 2005 paper consisted of a stepwise procedure starting with the prediction of violence followed by the prediction of homicide offenders among the violent youth. Similar analyses are described in Chap. 5. Fourth, predictors of homicide offenders were studied over a wide range of years prior to the commission of the murder, whereas predictors in this chapter were measured at the beginning of the PYS. Fifth, although the 2005 paper included behavioral and explanatory predictors, it did not clarify which prior offense types were most relevant for the prediction of homicide offenders.

Several key questions are addressed in this chapter. To what extent do factors measured in childhood (aged 7–13) predict convicted homicide offenders and to what extent can this prediction be made in the general population rather than in the population of violent boys? To what extent does a person's previous criminal history (up to age 14) predict convicted homicide offenders? These questions are important because they identify the early presence of risk factors several years prior to the murder taking place.

Risk factors are classified as explanatory or behavioral (Loeber and Farrington, 1998, pp. 105–108). Explanatory variables are those that clearly do not measure antisocial behavior. In contrast, behavioral variables (which include attitudinal variables) could reflect the boy's antisocial behavior. For example, a young mother and poor parental supervision were classified as explanatory variables, while truanting and suspension from school was classified as behavioral variables. In addition, criminal risk factors (prior offenses) are studied.

It is unclear which early explanatory or behavioral risk factors are the strongest predictors when the remaining risk factors are taken into account. For instance, are individual factors (such as callous-unemotional behavior, low level of guilt feelings, or hyperactivity–impulsivity–attention problems) stronger predictors than environmental factors (such as broken family,[1] a young mother, or living in a disadvantaged neighborhood) or the reverse? The 2005 paper summarized the best predictors into a risk score, but the question is now whether a dose–response relationship exists between the number of explanatory risk factors in *childhood* in the whole sample and the probability of later homicide offending.

Another inquiry focuses on early behavioral predictors of convicted homicide offenders. We are interested in identifying disruptive and delinquent behaviors occurring in childhood which predict later homicide offenders, and possibly are the most relevant for the early behavioral development of violence. For example, we need to know to what extent more serious behaviors (such as serious forms of delinquency or cruelty to people), that usually occur later in the developmental sequence leading to violence (Loeber et al., 1993), are better predictors of homicide offenders than less serious behaviors, such as truancy. Since many less and more serious forms of problem behaviors often occur in the company of peers, there is a need to know the extent to which peer factors (such as peer delinquency and having bad friends) add to the prediction of homicide offenders. Finally, because most of the convicted homicide offenders in the PYS were African American, and because African American boys tend to have more risk factors than Caucasian boys, it is important to know whether race predicts convicted homicide offenders once earlier risk factors are taken into account.

The identification of behavioral predictors that best predict convicted homicide offenders does not clarify which specific offenses committed during childhood and early adolescence are good predictors. Here the inquiry focuses on both self-reported offending and official reports of delinquent acts up to age 14, thus before the commission of any murder (the first homicide offender committed his crime at age 15). Once the answer to this question has been obtained, we also want to know to what extent a combination of explanatory, behavioral, and criminal risk factors measured up to age 14 improves on the accuracy of the prediction of convicted homicide offenders. We are also interested in assessing the accuracy of early screening instruments for homicide offending based on explanatory, behavioral, and criminal factors.

Most of the analyses in this chapter focus on convicted homicide offenders. However, we also investigate the extent to which individuals arrested for homicide but not convicted (called homicide arrestees) share the same childhood risk factors as convicted homicide offenders.

In summary, the key questions addressed in this chapter are as follows:

- To what extent did homicide offenders engage in antisocial and delinquent behavior earlier in life?
- Which explanatory, behavioral, and criminal risk factors predict homicide offenders out of a community sample up to 22 years later?

---

[1] This construct was formerly called "one or no biological parents in home" (Loeber et al., 2008a).

- To what extent can convicted homicide offenders be predicted based on a combination of explanatory, behavioral, and criminal risk factors?
- Is there a dose–response relationship between the number of risk factors and the probability of becoming a homicide offender?
- Are homicide offenders predominantly psychopaths?
- Are racial differences in the prevalence of homicide offenders attributable to racial differences in early risk factors?

Measurement of Childhood Risk Factors

This chapter compares childhood risk factors measured in the screening and first follow-up assessments (in 1987–1988) with later information about convicted homicide offenders.

The 21 explanatory risk factors were as follows (for more information about all these factors, see Table 2.3):

Child: Lack of guilt, HIA (hyperactivity–impulsivity–attention deficit), old for the grade (has been held back), low academic achievement (both according to the California Achievement Test and according to mother–teacher ratings), depressed mood, callous-unemotional (based on Frick, O'Brien, Wootton, & McBurnett, 1994).

Parental: Young mother (a teenager when the boy was born), father behavior problems (father seeking help for behavior problems; rated by the mother, so available for all fathers whether present or absent), parent substance use.

Child-Rearing: Poor parental supervision, physical punishment by the mother, poor parent–boy communication.

Socioeconomic: Low socioeconomic status (the Hollingshead measure, based on parental education and occupational prestige), family on welfare, broken family, large family size, small house, unemployed mother.

Neighborhood: Bad neighborhood (both according to 1990 census data and according to mother ratings).

These were derived from the 40 distinct explanatory factors described by Loeber et al. (1998a, Chap. 5) excluding those not known for all three cohorts, those with a large amount of missing data (e.g., variables referring to the operative father or to the mother–father relationship), and those not strongly related to delinquency in 1987–1988 [odds ratio (OR)<2.0]. Some variables were added because they were related to violence (OR≥2.0) in Farrington, Loeber, and Stouthamer-Loeber (2003). Most variables were based on interviews with mothers, in a few cases supplemented by data from boys. More information about all these variables can be found in Loeber et al. (1998a), Loeber et al. (2003), and Loeber, Farrington, Stouthamer-Loeber, and White (2008).

The most contentious variable was peer delinquency. We classified this as a behavioral variable because three-quarters of the delinquent acts committed by the boys were committed with their peers. Because of this, boys who had committed delinquent acts usually had delinquent peers. Also, Farrington, Loeber, Yin, and Anderson (2002) found that peer delinquency was the strongest correlate of a boy's delinquency in between-individual correlations (both measured at the same time) but did not predict a boy's later delinquency within individuals. They concluded that peer delinquency was not a cause of a boy's delinquency but, as recorded in self-reports, measured the same underlying construct as delinquency. In contrast, poor parental supervision was correlated with delinquency between individuals and predicted delinquency within individuals.

The 19 behavioral risk factors measured in 1987–1988 and used in this chapter were as follows:

Child Behavior: Serious delinquency (based on self-, parent- and teacher-report), covert behavior (concealing, manipulative, untrustworthy), physical aggression, nonphysical aggression, cruel to people, runs away, disruptive behavior disorder diagnosis (according to the Revised Diagnostic Interview Schedule for Children: Costello, Edelbrock, Kalas, Kessler, & Klaric, 1982), high (above-average) screening risk score.

Child Attitude: Positive attitude to delinquency, positive attitude to substance use.

Parental: Bad relationship with parent, counter control (the bad behavior of the boy inhibits parental attempts at socialization).

Peer: Peer delinquency, bad friends, bad relationship with peers.

School: Suspended, truant, negative attitude to school, low school motivation.

These were derived from the 25 correlates of delinquency described by Loeber et al. (1998a, Chap. 5), with exclusion rules similar to those used with explanatory variables.

More information about all these variables can be found in Loeber et al. (1998a, 2003, 2008). In addition, race (African American or Caucasian) was included in the analysis.

For the present analyses, the explanatory and behavioral risk factors were dichotomized within each cohort into, as far as possible, the "worst" quarter of males (e.g., the quarter with the lowest attainment or poorest supervision) vs. the remainder. This dichotomization fostered a "risk factor" approach and made it easy to study the cumulative effects of several risk factors. It also made all variables directly comparable, by equating sensitivity of measurement, and permitted the use of the odds ratio as a measure of strength of relationship, which has many advantages (Fleiss, 1981). In the Pittsburgh Youth Study, conclusions about the most important explanatory variables for delinquency were not greatly affected by using dichotomous as opposed to continuous variables or by different dichotomization splits (Farrington & Loeber, 2000b).

Dichotomizing the variables within each cohort made all the cohorts comparable and made it possible to combine them. Arguably, the quarter of the youngest cohort with the poorest parental supervision (for example) were comparable to the quarter of the oldest cohort with the poorest parental supervision, even though the absolute levels of parental supervision were different in all three cohorts.

This chapter contrasts 37 convicted homicide offenders with 1,406 control boys. The first homicide offense was committed at age 15. Therefore, one boy who emigrated permanently before this age and four boys who died before age 15 were excluded, since they were not realistically at risk of offending. The 33 arrested but not convicted homicide offenders were also excluded, as were 36 homicide victims who were neither convicted nor arrested (two convicted offenders and one arrested offender were also homicide victims).

Explanatory Predictors

The first question concerned the explanatory risk factors measured between ages 7 and 13 which predicted convicted homicide offenders in the full population of young males. Table 4.1 summarizes the results. For ease of exposition, retrospective percentages are presented. For example, Table 4.1 shows that 89% of offenders, compared with 62% of controls, came from a broken home (OR = 5.0, CI 1.8–14.3; confidence intervals are large because of the small number of homicide offenders). In other words, nine out of ten convicted homicide offenders had a missing biological parent (usually the father) by the first year of the study.

Nine of the 21 explanatory factors significantly predicted convicted homicide offenders: broken home, a bad neighborhood (according to Census data), the family on welfare, a young mother, old for the grade (held back), an unemployed mother, lack of guilt, behavior problems of the father, and low socioeconomic status (Table 4.1). Hyperactivity–impulsivity–attention deficit was on the borderline of statistical significance (OR = 2.0, CI = 0.99–4.2). The strongest predictors were broken home (OR = 5.0), living in a bad neighborhood (OR = 3.9), family on welfare (OR = 3.2), and a young mother (OR = 3.1). Heide (1999) also argued that young homicide offenders tended to come from broken homes. The results show that the strongest explanatory predictors were environmental factors and that individual factors tended to be somewhat weaker (e.g., old for the grade, OR = 2.9; lack of guilt, OR = 2.4).

Table 4.1 Explanatory predictors of convicted homicide offenders

	% of controls (1,406)	% of offenders (37)	Odds ratio	Partial OR	p
Broken family	62	89	5.0*	–	–
Bad neighborhood (C)	32	65	3.9*	3.2	.004
Family on welfare	43	71	3.2*	–	–
Young mother	21	45	3.1*	2.5	.016
Old for the grade	25	49	2.9*	–	–
Unemployed mother	25	45	2.6*	1.9	.081
Lack of guilt	24	43	2.4*	–	–
Father behavior problems	17	32	2.4*	–	–
Low socioeconomic status	26	43	2.2*	2.0	.064
HIA	17	30	2.0	–	–

Notes: C census, *HIA* hyperactivity–impulsivity–attention deficit, OR odds ratio
*$p < .05$

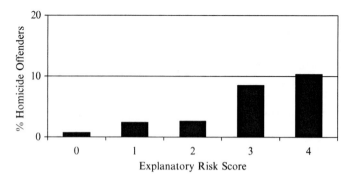

Fig. 4.1 Explanatory risk score predicting convicted homicide offenders

Explanatory Risk Score. A logistic regression analysis was carried out to investigate which of the nine significant predictors of homicide offenders were independent predictors. Four variables were significant or nearly significant in a stepwise analysis: a bad neighborhood (likelihood ratio chi-squared or LRCS = 15.05, $p = <.0001$), a young mother (LRCS = 6.92, $p = .009$), low socioeconomic status (LRCS = 3.84, $p = .050$), and an unemployed mother (LRCS = 2.96, $p = .086$). In the final model, the partial odds ratios were 3.2 for a bad neighborhood, 2.5 for a young mother, 2.0 for low socioeconomic status, and 1.9 for an unemployed mother (see Table 4.1).

An explanatory risk score was calculated for each boy based on the number of these four risk factors that he possessed. Figure 4.1 shows that the higher the explanatory risk score, the higher the percentage of homicide offenders. For example, 0.7% of boys with none of these four risk factors were homicide offenders, compared with 8.5% of boys with three risk factors and 10.3% of boys with all four risk factors. Therefore, there was significant predictability but also a high false-positive rate. Retrospectively, 15 of the 37 homicide offenders (41%) were among the 12% of boys with three or four of these risk factors (Fig. 4.1). Comparing boys with 0–2 risk factors with those with 3–4 risk factors produced an OR = 5.4 (CI = 2.8–10.7); comparing boys with 0–3 risk factors with those with four risk factors produced an OR = 4.7 (CI = 1.3–16.1). However, the main measure of predictive accuracy that is used in this book is the area under the ROC curve (AUC), which in this example was .735 (SD = .042). This value is statistically significant, because it is more than 2 standard deviations above the chance value of .50. In general, an AUC value of .7 or greater indicates good predictability. The best-fitting ROC was calculated by maximum likelihood techniques, assuming underlying normal distributions, using the ROCFIT software of Charles E. Metz. The interpretation of the AUC is as follows: If we choose a homicide offender at random, and he happens to have a score of Y, and we choose a control at random, and he happens to have a score of X, the AUC is the probability that Y will be greater than X. Therefore, in 73.5% of cases, the homicide offender would have a higher risk score than the control.

Why Does Race Predict Homicide Offenders?

As found in many other studies (Centers for Disease Control, 2008), African American boys were more likely to be convicted homicide offenders than were Caucasian boys: 86% of offenders were African American, compared with 54% of controls (OR=5.4, CI=2.1–13.8). The question that we raise is: *Are racial differences in the prevalence of homicide offenders attributable to racial differences in early risk factors?*

It is plausible to suggest that race predicts convicted homicide offenders because African American and Caucasian boys differ on predictive risk factors. According to this hypothesis, race should not predict homicide offenders after controlling for other predictive explanatory risk factors. Indeed, after entering the nine significant explanatory risk factors in a logistic regression analysis, race did not significantly predict convicted homicide offenders.

It might be concluded that race predicted convicted homicide offenders primarily because of racial differences in exposure to risk factors known to predict murder. Of the nine explanatory risk factors, the strongest correlates with race were: broken home (81% of African Americans vs. 42% of Caucasians; OR=5.9, CI=4.7–7.5), the family on welfare (61% of African Americans vs. 23% of Caucasians: OR=5.1, CI=4.0–6.4), a bad neighborhood (65% of African Americans vs. 32% of Caucasians: OR=3.9, CI=2.0–7.7), and a young mother (30% of African Americans vs. 13% of Caucasians: OR=2.9, CI=2.2–3.8). It is possible that African American boys were more likely to be convicted homicide offenders because they differed from Caucasian boys in their exposure to these socioeconomic risk factors.

Behavioral Predictors

We now turn to behavioral predictors of homicide, which include attitudinal factors as well. The results show that 11 of the 19 factors significantly predicted convicted homicide offenders. These included suspended from school, a high (above-average) screening risk score, a positive attitude to delinquency, disruptive behavior disorder, serious delinquency, peer delinquency, a positive attitude to substance use, covert behavior (concealing, manipulative, untrustworthy), cruelty to people, bad friends, and truancy (Table 4.2). The strongest predictor was suspended from school: 78% of homicide offenders were suspended compared with 43% of controls (OR=4.9, CI=2.2–10.7).

Behavioral Risk Score. A logistic regression analysis was carried out to investigate which of the 11 significant behavioral predictors of homicide offenders were independent predictors. Four variables were significant or nearly significant in a stepwise analysis: a positive attitude to delinquency (LRCS=16.01, $p<.0001$), suspended from school (LRCS=15.10, $p=.0001$), disruptive behavior disorder (LRCS=6.52, $p=.011$), and, marginally, a high screening risk score (LRCS=3.51, $p=.061$).

Table 4.2 Behavioral predictors of convicted homicide offenders

	% of controls (1,406)	% of offenders (37)	Odds ratio	Partial OR	p
Suspended	43	78	4.9*	2.9	.012
High-risk score	49	81	4.4*	2.2	.076
Positive attitude to delinquency	23	54	3.9*	2.9	.002
Disruptive behavior disorder	23	51	3.5*	2.1	.038
Serious delinquency	29	57	3.3*	–	–
Peer delinquency	24	49	3.0*	–	–
Positive attitude to substance use	24	46	2.7*	–	–
Covert behavior	24	46	2.7*	–	–
Cruel to people	24	43	2.4*	–	–
Bad friends	25	41	2.0*	–	–
Truant	38	54	1.9*	–	–

*Notes: *p<.05; OR* odds ratio

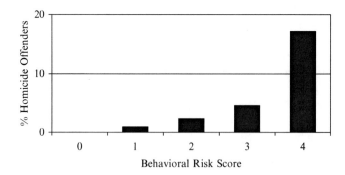

Fig. 4.2 Behavioral risk score predicting convicted homicide offenders

In the final model, the partial odds ratios were 2.9 for suspended from school, 2.9 for a positive attitude to delinquency, 2.2 for a high screening risk score, and 2.1 for disruptive behavior disorder.

A behavioral risk score was then calculated for each boy based on the number of these four risk factors that he possessed. Figure 4.2 shows a dose–response relationship between the risk score and the probability of becoming a homicide offender: the higher the behavior risk score, the higher the percentage of homicide offenders. For example, 0.7% of boys with none of these four risk factors were homicide offenders, compared with 17.1% of boys with four risk factors. Again, there was significant predictability but also a high false-positive rate. Prospectively, 22 of the 290 worst boys (8%) were convicted homicide offenders. Retrospectively, 22 of the 37 homicide offenders (59%) were among the one-fifth of the boys with three or more of these risk factors. Comparing boys with 0–2 risk factors with those with 3–4 risk factors produced an OR=11.1 (CI=3.2–12.2); comparing boys with 0–3 risk factors with those with four risk factors produced an OR=6.2

(CI = 5.3–23.3). The AUC = .773 (SD = .044). Not surprisingly, the behavioral factors predicted convicted homicide offenders more strongly than did the explanatory factors.

The Use of the Screening Risk Score in Estimating True Prediction

While the ability of the explanatory and behavioral risk scores to predict convicted homicide offenders is quite impressive, it is possible that predictive efficiency is overestimated in these analyses. This is because the risk score is calculated in light of knowledge about which risk factors were the best predictors of homicide offenders. In order to derive a more accurate estimate of predictive efficiency, we turned to the screening risk scores for each of the PYS participants. These were based on the initial contacts at ages 7–13 with the boy, his parent, and his teacher, before any later outcomes were known.

The screening risk score was based on the following 21 behaviors: attack, run away, set fires, steal from places other than the home, truancy, vandalism, steal from car, robbery, steal bicycle, shoplift, steal car, attack with a weapon, gang fight, hit/hurt teacher, hit/hurt parent, joyride, burglary, arrested, liquor use, sniff glue, and marijuana use (see Loeber et al., 1998a, p. 50). Each boy was scored according to the number of these 21 behaviors that he had committed. The average score was 2.1 for the youngest cohort (age 7), 3.2 for the middle cohort (age 10), and 4.2 for the oldest cohort (age 13).

For the present analyses, each boy was given a Z-score (with a mean of 0 and a standard deviation of 1) relative to his cohort. Therefore, all the cohort scores were comparable. We divided these Z-scores into seven categories and show how they predicted convicted homicide offenders. Figure 4.3 shows that the higher the Z-score, the higher the probability of becoming a homicide offender (a stepwise function). For example, 8.3% of boys with the highest Z-scores (at least 2 standard deviations above the mean) were convicted, compared with 0.5% of boys with the lowest Z-scores. Retrospectively, 19 of the 37 homicide offenders (51%) were among the

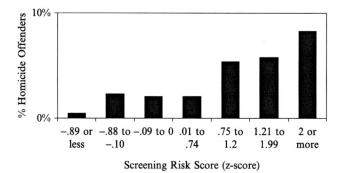

Fig. 4.3 Screening risk score predicting convicted homicide offenders

one-fifth of the boys in the top three categories (Z-score .75 or greater). Comparing boys in these categories with the remainder, OR=4.0 (CI=2.1–7.7). The AUC was .709 (SD=.041).

Comparing results from the screening risk score with those from the behavioral risk score, the AUC decreased from .773 to .709, and the comparable OR (based on the highest one-fifth of boys) decreased from 6.2 to 4.0. Part of this decrease is attributable to the more limited predictor (based on only one variable rather than several different variables) but another part probably reflects the overestimation of predictive efficiency by the behavioral risk score. It is reasonable to suggest that an unbiased AUC based on a behavioral risk score might be of the order of .72–.75, that an unbiased OR might be of the order of 5, and that about 7% of the worst one-fifth of the sample might become convicted homicide offenders.

Homicide Arrestees

As mentioned, 33 boys were arrested for homicide but not convicted (including four boys who were arrested for attempted murder and one convicted for attempted murder). *To what extent were the homicide arrestees exposed to the same childhood risk factors as the convicted homicide offenders?* The answer was: Not a lot.

Out of 40 (explanatory and behavioral) childhood risk factors, 16 significantly predicted the 33 homicide arrestees (compared with 21 which significantly predicted the 37 convicted homicide offenders). However, there was not a great deal of overlap between the predictors of homicide arrestees and the predictors of convicted homicide offenders: only 9 of the 21 significant predictors of homicide offenders were among the 16 significant predictors of homicide arrestees.

The next questions that we raised were: *What are the best predictors of the convicted plus arrested homicide offenders (out of all violent boys)?* And *How do these differ from the strongest predictors of the convicted homicide offenders?* Table 4.3 shows the nine overlapping risk factors and also the other seven significant predictors of homicide arrestees. The homicide arrestees were even more likely to be African American boys than were the homicide offenders: 31 of the 33 homicide arrestees (94%) were African American, compared with 54% of the 1,406 controls (OR=13.0, CI=3.1– 54.5). It is possible that African American boys are more likely than Caucasian boys to be arrested when they are in fact innocent, or alternatively it is possible that African American boys are more effective than Caucasian boys in terrorizing witnesses so that there is insufficient evidence for a trial.

Aside from African American race, the strongest predictor of homicide arrestees was truancy: 79% of homicide arrestees were truant, compared with 38% of controls (OR=6.2, CI=2.7–14.3). Truancy was only a weak predictor of convicted offenders (OR=1.9, CI=1.0–3.8). It may be that the homicide arrestees, rather than spending time in school, were hanging out more on the street where arrests are more likely to take place. Other strong common predictors of homicide arrestees and

Table 4.3 Predictors of arrested vs. convicted homicide offenders

	% of controls (1,406)	% of arrested (33)	Odds ratio arrested	Odds ratio convicted
Predictors of arrested and of convicted offenders				
Truancy	38	79	6.2*	1.9*
Peer delinquency	24	50	3.2*	3.0*
Broken family	62	84	3.2*	5.0*
Serious delinquency	29	55	3.0*	3.3*
Suspended	43	68	2.8*	4.9*
Old for the grade	25	48	2.8*	2.9*
Cruel to people	24	42	2.3*	2.4*
Disruptive behavior disorder	23	39	2.1*	3.5*
African American	54	94	13.0*	5.4*
Predictors of arrested but not of convicted offenders				
Low achievement (CAT)	24	48	3.0*	1.3
Low achievement (PT)	24	48	3.0*	1.3
Bad neighborhood (P)	24	48	2.9*	1.3
Low school motivation	37	63	2.9*	1.8
Nonphysical aggression	25	45	2.5*	1.8
Poor communication	26	42	2.1*	1.6
Bad relationship with peers	26	42	2.1*	1.6

Notes: *$p<.05$, *CAT* California Achievement Test, *P* parent, *T* teacher, *C* census, *OR* odds ratio. Predictors of convicted but not of arrested offenders: Bad neighborhood (C), family on welfare, young mother (OR = 2.0 for arrested), unemployed mother, lack of guilt (OR = 2.0 for arrested), father behavior problems, low socioeconomic status, high screening risk score, positive attitude to delinquency, positive attitude to substance use, covert behavior, bad friends

convicted offenders were peer delinquency, broken home, serious delinquency, suspended from school, and old for the grade.

The strongest unique predictors of homicide arrestees were low school achievement (both according to the California Achievement Test and parent–teacher ratings) and low school motivation, which are factors strongly associated with truancy. The homicide arrestees also tended to reside in a bad neighborhood (according to the parent) and were high on nonphysical aggression. In contrast, the strongest predictors of convicted offenders (but not of homicide arrestees) were a high screening risk score, a positive attitude to delinquency, living in a bad neighborhood (according to the census), the family on welfare, a young mother (although the OR for homicide arrestees was nearly significant at 2.0), a positive attitude to substance use, and engaging in covert behavior.

In summary, there was some tendency for behavioral factors to be more characteristic of homicide arrestees and for socioeconomic factors to be more characteristic of convicted homicide offenders. The behavioral factors that were more characteristic of homicide arrestees included truancy, low school achievement, low school motivation, and nonphysical aggression. The socioeconomic factors that were more characteristic of convicted homicide offenders included a broken family, the family on welfare, a young mother, an unemployed mother, and low socioeconomic status.

Offending at a Young Age of Convicted Homicide Offenders

It is believed that most homicide offenders were violent earlier in life (Loeber et al., 2005a) and also committed many other illegal activities (see, e.g., Brodie, Daday, Crandall, Sklar, & Jost, 2006; Cook & Laub, 1998; Cook, Ludwig, & Braga, 2005). To what extent can convicted homicide offenders be predicted on the basis of their prior criminal histories? What types of crimes are precursors to homicide offending? In order to investigate these questions, three sources of information about prior offending were used: self-reports, convictions, and arrests. Only crimes committed up to age 14 were studied, to ensure that all prior crimes occurred before the first homicide conviction. Thus, the following information pertains to the early criminal careers of convicted homicide offenders. As before, 37 convicted homicide offenders were compared with 1,406 control boys.

The following categories of self-reported crimes were studied: robbery, aggravated assault, gang fighting, weapon carrying (violence), burglary, theft of vehicle, theft from person, theft from a car, shoplifting, other theft, receiving, arson, vandalism (property), drug selling, hard drug use, marijuana use (drugs), minor fraud/avoid paying. Heide (1999) concluded that young homicide offenders tended to have a prior history of drug and alcohol abuse. In addition, we studied three other categories of substance use: drunk in public, alcohol use, and tobacco use. Alcohol use and intoxication are particularly associated with violence (White, Jackson, & Loeber, 2009). The following categories of arrests and convictions were studied: robbery, aggravated assault, simple assault, threats, weapons, serious sex offenses (violence), burglary, theft of vehicle, larceny, receiving, vandalism (property), drugs, mischief/disorder, other/conspiracy (other crimes). The other/conspiracy category is labeled because the "other" category in the records included primarily criminal conspiracy offenses (where two or more people were involved in planning a crime together).

Table 4.4 shows the extent to which self-reported offenses before age 15 predicted convicted homicide offenders. The strongest predictor was vehicle theft, closely followed by weapon carrying. Other strong predictors were the total violence score, minor fraud (avoid paying), robbery, the total theft score, drug selling, vandalism, and theft from a car (all ORs greater than 3.0). The surprising finding is that, while the commission of violent and drug crimes did predict later homicide offending, so did the commission of a range of other property crimes and even minor deviance such as tobacco use. These results suggest that homicide offenders at a young age were already versatile offenders (i.e., engaging in a large variety of different offense types) prior to committing murder. Contrary to our expectations, several self-reported forms of substance use (hard drug use, marijuana use, drunk in public, and alcohol use) did not significantly predict later homicide offending.

How do convictions for delinquency in the juvenile court compare to self-reported delinquency as predictors of homicide offending? Table 4.5 shows the extent to which convictions up to age 14 predicted convicted homicide offenders. In total, 21 of the 37 offenders (57%) were convicted up to age 14, compared with 17%

Table 4.4 Prediction of convicted homicide offenders by self-reported delinquency up to age 14

Offenses	% of controls (1,406)	% of convicted (37)	Odds ratio
Violence			
Robbery	3	11	4.1*
Aggravated assault	13	24	2.2*
Gang fight	23	41	2.3*
Violence (3)	28	62	4.2*
Weapon carrying	39	76	4.8*
Property			
Burglary	13	30	2.8*
Vehicle theft	12	41	4.9*
Theft from person	7	3	0.4
Theft from car	13	32	3.2*
Theft (4)	27	57	3.6*
Shoplifting	46	68	2.5*
Other theft	44	59	1.9
Receiving	15	16	1.1
Arson	12	16	1.4
Vandalism	53	78	3.2*
Drug			
Drug selling	8	22	3.4*
Hard drug use	6	12	2.4
Marijuana use	15	27	2.0
Drug (3)	19	35	2.3*
Other deviance			
Minor fraud	46	78	4.2*
Drunk in public	9	14	1.7
Alcohol use	63	73	1.6
Tobacco use	34	51	2.1*

Notes: Violence (3) is any of the three prior violence offenses
Theft (4) is any of the four prior property offenses
Drug (3) is any of the three prior drug offenses
*$p < .05$

of the 1,406 controls (OR = 6.4, CI = 3.3–12.5). The types of crimes that most strongly predicted later homicide offenses were weapons offenses, robbery, simple assault, other/conspiracy, total violence, and receiving stolen property. While all types of violent crimes predicted later homicide offending, so did all types of property crimes, reinforcing the notion that the early offense patterns of homicide offenders are versatile rather than specialized. However, because of the low prevalence, drug convictions did not significantly predict later homicide offending.

How do predictors of homicide offenders compare as a function of official records of conviction and self-reported delinquency? Table 4.5 shows that conviction for different forms of violence is a stronger predictor of homicide than is self-reported violence. Also, conviction for receiving stolen goods, an indication of participation in the illegal economy, is a strong predictor of homicide offenders (OR = 6.8, $p < .05$), but its self-reported equivalent was not (OR = 1.1, n.s.).

Table 4.5 Prediction of convicted homicide offenders by convictions up to age 14

Crime	% of controls (1,406)	% of convicted (37)	Odds ratio
Violence			
Robbery	1	11	9.9*
Aggravated assault	3	14	5.9*
Simple assault	3	24	9.7*
Violence (3)	5	30	7.5*
Threats	2	11	5.0*
Weapons	0	5	13.3*
Sex	2	8	5.1*
Property			
Burglary	4	13	3.4*
Vehicle theft	5	16	3.6*
Larceny	5	22	5.8*
Theft (3)	10	32	4.6*
Receiving	6	30	6.8*
Vandalism	5	16	4.1*
Other			
Drug	1	3	2.6
Mischief/disorder	3	5	2.0
Other/conspiracy	11	51	8.5*
Any conviction	17	57	6.4*

Notes: Violence (3) is any of the three prior violence offenses
Theft (3) is any of the three prior property offenses
*$p < .05$

Table 4.6 shows the extent to which arrests up to age 14 (which were more numerous than convictions) predicted convicted homicide offenders. In total, 26 of the 37 offenders (70%) were arrested up to age 14, compared with 28% of the 1,406 controls (OR = 6.2, CI = 3.0–12.6). The types of crimes that most strongly predicted later homicide offenses were different forms of violence, including aggravated assault, weapons, other/conspiracy, simple assault, robbery, combined violence, and threats. All of the property arrests were significant predictors of later homicide offenders, although less strongly so than for violent arrests. Again, because of the low prevalence before age 15, drug arrests did not significantly predict later homicide offenders.

Criminal Risk Score. Logistic regression analyses were carried out to investigate which types of prior offenses up to age 14 independently predicted later convictions for homicide. Separate analyses were carried out for self-reports, convictions, and arrests. All significant offense variables were entered in the regressions. Table 4.7 shows the results. Self-reported vehicle theft, weapon carrying, and minor fraud (avoid paying) independently predicted later homicide offending. Convictions for other/conspiracy and simple assault were also independent predictors, as were arrests for other/conspiracy, weapons, and simple assault.

Table 4.6 Prediction of convicted homicide offenders by arrests up to age 14

	% of controls (1,406)	% of convicted (37)	Odds ratio
Violence			
Robbery	3	16	6.1*
Aggravated assault	4	24	7.6*
Simple assault	7	32	6.6*
Violence (3)	11	43	6.0*
Threats	6	27	5.8*
Weapons	6	32	7.0*
Sex	3	11	3.9*
Property			
Burglary	7	16	2.6*
Vehicle theft	7	18	3.0*
Larceny	10	22	2.6*
Theft (3)	15	32	2.7*
Receiving	10	30	3.7*
Vandalism	9	27	3.9*
Other			
Drug	2	3	1.3
Mischief/disorder	6	11	2.0
Other/conspiracy	17	59	6.9*
Any arrest	28	70	6.2*

Notes: Violence (3) is any of the three prior violence offenses
Theft (3) is any of the three prior property offenses
*$p < .05$

All of these eight variables were then entered into a final logistic regression analysis to establish the independent criminal predictors from all of the self-report, conviction, and arrest information before age 15. The bottom of Table 4.7 shows the results. Five variables were significant independent predictors: other/conspiracy convictions, self-reports of weapon carrying, arrests for weapons and simple assault, and self-reports of minor fraud (avoiding paying).

A criminal risk score was then calculated based on the number of these five risk factors that each boy possessed. Figure 4.4 shows a dose–response relationship between the criminal risk score and the probability of becoming a homicide offender: the higher that score, the higher the percentage of homicide offenders. A total of 46 boys (3%) possessed four or five risk factors, and 10 of them were convicted (22%), compared with 2% of the remaining 1,397 who were known. However, only 10 of the 37 offenders (27%) were identified by this cut-off point (OR = 14.1; CI = 6.3–31.3). A total of 155 boys (11%) possessed three, four, or five of the risk factors, and 22 of them were convicted (14%), compared with 1% of the remaining 1,288 boys (OR = 14.0; CI = 7.1–27.7). This cut-off point identified 59% of the homicide offenders. Perhaps not surprisingly, the AUC of .837 (SD = .035) for criminal risk factors was much higher than for the explanatory or behavioral risk factors (.735 and .773, respectively).

Table 4.7 Logistic regression analyses predicting convicted homicide offenders

Based on:	LRCS	p	Partial OR	p
Self-reports				
Vehicle theft	18.09	.0001	2.6	.010
Weapon carrying	10.66	.001	2.8	.015
Minor fraud	4.35	.037	2.4	.047
Convictions				
Other/conspiracy	35.20	.0001	6.1	.0001
Simple assault	5.56	.018	3.2	.014
Arrests				
Other/conspiracy	31.37	.0001	4.0	.0003
Weapons	10.07	.002	3.4	.002
Simple assault	4.24	.040	2.4	.034
All				
Other/conspiracy (C)	34.37	.0001	3.7	.0005
Weapon carrying (S)	12.83	.0003	2.8	.013
Weapons (A)	8.27	.004	3.0	.007
Simple assault (A)	4.72	.030	2.6	.019
Minor fraud (S)	4.10	.043	2.3	.054

Notes: (S) self-reports, *(C)* convictions, *(A)* arrests
LRCS Likelihood ratio chi-squared, *OR* odds ratio

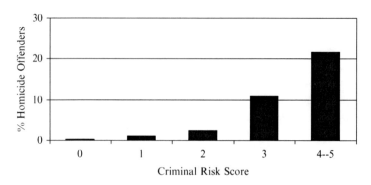

Fig. 4.4 Criminal risk score predicting convicted homicide offenders

The Use of Arrests in Estimating Overprediction

As before, it might be argued that predictive efficiency is overestimated in this analysis of criminal risk scores, because the constituent variables are chosen in light of knowledge about which are the best predictors. In order to produce a more realistic assessment of predictive efficiency, we looked solely at the number of arrests up to age 14, as an unbiased measure of criminal risk.

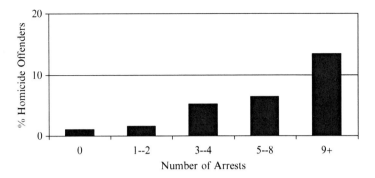

Fig. 4.5 Number of arrests up to age 14 predicting convicted homicide offenders

Figure 4.5 shows a dose–response relationship between the number of arrests up to age 14 and the probability of becoming a homicide offender: The higher the arrest number, the higher the percentage of homicide offenders. Of 97 boys with nine or more arrests, 13 (13%) were convicted, compared with 2% of the 1,346 boys with fewer arrests (OR = 8.5; CI = 4.2–17.3). However, only 13 of the 37 offenders (35%) were identified by this cutoff point. Of 189 boys with five or more arrests, 19 (10%) were convicted, compared with 1% of the 1,254 boys with fewer arrests (OR = 7.7; CI = 3.9–14.9). This cutoff point identified 19 of the 37 offenders (51%).

Comparing results from the number of arrests with those from the criminal risk score, the AUC decreased from .837 to .794 (SD = .046), and the most comparable OR decreased from 14.0 to 7.7. Part of this decrease is attributable to the more limited predictor (based on number of arrests only, not on types of offenses or on convictions or self-reports) and another part probably reflects the overestimation of predictive efficiency by the criminal risk score. It is reasonable to suggest that an unbiased AUC based on a criminal risk score might be of the order of .81–.82, that an unbiased OR might be of the order of 10, and that about 11–12% of the worst one-eighth of the sample might become convicted homicide offenders.

Final, Integrated Prediction of Homicide Offenders

In the final exercise to predict convicted homicide offenders, all the significant, independently predictive risk factors (explanatory, behavioral, and criminal) from Tables 4.1, 4.2, and 4.7 were entered into a logistic regression analysis. This included the following explanatory factors: a bad neighborhood, a young mother, low socioeconomic status, and an unemployed mother; the following behavioral factors: a positive attitude to delinquency, suspended from school, disruptive behavior disorder, and high screening risk score; the following self-reported offending types: weapon carrying and minor fraud; the following conviction type: other/conspiracy; and the following arrest types: weapons and simple assault.

Table 4.8 Final logistic regression analysis predicting convicted homicide offenders

Predictors	LRCS	p	Partial OR	p
Other/conspiracy (conviction)	31.05	.0001	3.9	.0008
Suspended	16.83	.0001	3.9	.008
Weapon carrying (self-report)	10.87	.001	3.0	.011
Simple assault (arrest)	7.32	.007	3.1	.010
Positive attitude to delinquency	6.18	.013	2.4	.025
Bad neighborhood (census)	4.91	.027	2.3	.033
Young mother	3.50	.062	2.1	.057

Notes: LRCS likelihood ratio chi-squared, *OR* odds ratio

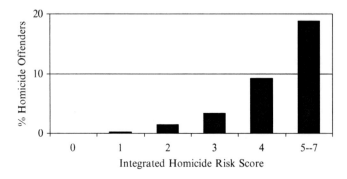

Fig. 4.6 Integrated homicide risk score predicting convicted homicide offenders

Table 4.8 shows the results of the final logistic regression analysis based on the above mentioned 13 risk factors. Seven risk factors independently predicted convicted homicide offenders: conviction for other/conspiracy, suspended from school, self-reported weapon carrying, arrest for simple assault, positive attitude to delinquency, living in a bad neighborhood, and a young mother. Thus, among the best predictors were prior delinquent acts (other crimes/conspiracy, simple assault, weapon carrying), antisocial attitude (favoring delinquency), family disadvantage (a young mother), and living in a disadvantaged neighborhood when young. All of these factors were recorded up to age 14, indicating that these independent risk factors are already in place in different domains of functioning (individual, family, and neighborhood) well before the commission of murder.

Integrated Homicide Risk Score. How well did the seven most important risk factors predict homicide and did they add up in a dose–response manner? Figure 4.6 shows an increasing dose–response relationship between the integrated homicide risk score and the probability of becoming a homicide offender. None of the 282 young males with no risk factors was convicted of homicide, compared with 13 of the 69 boys with 5, 6, or 7 risk factors (19%) (OR=13.2; CI=6.7–26.2). The AUC was .870

(SD = .029), which was substantially higher than the earlier AUC's for explanatory risk factors (AUC = .735), behavioral risk factors (AUC = .773), and criminal risk factors (AUC = .837). Of the 69 young males (5%) who scored 5–7 or higher, 13 (19%) were convicted, compared with 24 (2%) of the remaining 1,371 boys whose scores were known. This cutoff point identified only 35% of the offenders. Of the 178 young males (12%) who scored four or higher, 23 (13%) were convicted of homicide, compared with 14 (1%) of the remaining 1,262 boys (OR = 13.0; CI = 6.3–26.9). This cutoff point identified 62% of the convicted homicide offenders.

Overall, these are impressive results that show the considerable predictability of homicide offending. As we have demonstrated, the results may overestimate the true predictive efficacy because this scale was constructed and tested on the same people, rather than being validated on several independent samples. For that reason, this prediction scale needs to be applied to an independent sample sometime in the future for further validation. Nevertheless, the results suggest that possessing four of the seven risk factors listed in Fig. 4.6 by age 14 might be a useful means of predicting future homicide offenders. However, caution is needed in that the results fail to identify one third of the homicide offenders (false-negative rate = 38%), and there is substantial overprediction (false-positive rate = 87%).

Conclusions

We set out to undertake the very difficult task of predicting convicted homicide offenders in a general population sample of young males in public schools. This task was difficult because we wanted to predict the 2% of the population who had killed someone, and it was made even more difficult because we wanted to concentrate on risk factors measured relatively early in life, that is up to age 14, with many of the factors measured even as early as age 7 (in the youngest cohort). We set about this task by first examining explanatory factors by themselves, then behavioral factors, then prior offenses, and finally by integrating the preceding sets of risk factors. We compared 37 convicted homicide offenders with 1,406 controls.

It was noteworthy that the most important explanatory predictors of convicted homicide offenders were environmental and socioeconomic rather than individual factors: broken home, a bad neighborhood, the family on welfare, and a young mother. Similarly, the independent predictors were all socioeconomic: a bad neighborhood, a young mother, an unemployed mother, and low socioeconomic status of the family. While African American boys were more likely than Caucasian boys to be convicted homicide offenders, this was largely because they were more likely to possess socioeconomic risk factors such as (in particular) a broken home, the family on welfare, a bad neighborhood, and a young mother.

The most important behavioral risk factors that predicted convicted homicide offenders were suspended from school, disruptive behavior disorder, and a positive attitude to delinquency. Generally, behavioral risk factors were stronger predictors than were explanatory risk factors.

Prior criminal offenses up to age 14 were the most important risk factors for convicted homicide offenders. Not surprisingly, prior violence (especially assault and weapon carrying) was highly predictive. More surprisingly, prior property offenses (especially vehicle theft and minor fraud) were also highly predictive, as was criminal conspiracy. In general, the convicted homicide offenders tended to be versatile offenders up to age 14.

We also investigated the predictors of 33 homicide arrestees, but found that they were not very similar to the predictors of convicted homicide offenders. The most important early predictors of homicide arrestees tended to be school factors such as truancy, low school achievement, and low school motivation, rather than the kinds of socioeconomic factors that predicted convicted homicide offenders.

We now turn to the factors that were nonsignificant in the separate analyses and the integrated analyses. It was noteworthy that none of the parental child-rearing factors predicted convicted homicide offenders. There could be several reasons for this. First, other explanatory factors in the family environment appear to influence more who becomes a murderer, such having a young mother and living in a bad neighborhood. Second, prior research on this sample shows that the absence of violence (including homicide) is better predicted by the positive side of child-rearing practices (i.e., promotive factors), rather than the risk side of child-rearing practices predicting violence (Loeber, Farrington, Stouthamer-Loeber, & White, 2008). Another negative finding in the present results is that peer factors (peer delinquency according to the youth, and bad friends according to parents) did not independently predict homicide offenders in the final equation of the behavioral analyses. This finding is important, because it agrees with earlier analyses (Farrington, Loeber, Yin, & Anderson, 2002) indicating that peer factors probably reflect the same underlying construct as the participants' delinquency. Contrary to the conclusions of Heide (1999), low school achievement did not significantly predict convicted homicide offenders.

Another negative finding is that lack of guilt, cruelty to people, and callous-unemotional behavior, often thought to be early indicators of psychopathy, did not predict convicted homicide offenders. Thus, the results do not support the notion that early psychopathic features are related to homicide offending in this sample of predominantly street homicide offenders. This does not preclude the possibility that the four offenders who clearly were not street homicide offenders (mostly of Caucasian race) were more psychopathic, but their low number in this study precluded separate analyses. However, the follow-up data show that a proportion of the homicide offenders scored high enough in adulthood to qualify for the identification of psychopaths, and this is reported in Chap. 7. The results may indicate that the link between early signs of psychopathy in childhood and psychopathy in adulthood is not perfect, that psychopathy is less trait-like than is often presumed, and that psychopathic features may emerge in the course of delinquency careers, perhaps as a result of individuals' desensitization as a result of repeated violent offending.

On the positive side, the integrated analyses predicting convicted homicide offenders show that there is no single predictor as is often assumed, but that homicide offending is best predicted by a range of risk factors. This range includes explanatory and behavioral factors, and prior offenses. The final regression results show that independent predictors can be found among the explanatory environmental factors (a bad neighborhood and a young mother), the early manifestations of problem behavior (school suspension and a positive attitude to delinquency), and early versatile offense patterns, including self-reported weapon carrying, conviction for other/conspiracy offenses, and arrest for simple assault. The results support the notion that homicide offending is an outcome that is preceded by a history of disruptive, nondelinquent behavior, and delinquent acts. The fact that this history includes weapon carrying is significant, because the majority of the homicides were committed with a weapon, mostly a gun. The results also lend support to the notion that information from the police and courts can increase the predictability of homicide offending.

We carried out many analyses to assess how accurately convicted homicide offenders might be predicted in childhood using risk scores. There was a dose–response relationship: as the risk score increased, the probability of becoming a homicide offender increased, from less than 1% to 20% or so. Typically, it was possible to identify a high-risk group of about 15–20% of the sample. Out of this group about 8–14% became convicted homicide offenders. Therefore, false-positive rates were high. This high-risk group typically included half, or a little more than half, of all homicide offenders.

We dealt with the overprediction problem by investigating predictors that were not biased by the knowledge of who became convicted homicide offenders, namely the screening risk score and the number of arrests up to age 14. Our best estimate of predictive accuracy is that the AUC ranged from about .72–.75 for explanatory risk factors to .81–.82 for criminal risk factors. Therefore, homicide offenders were higher than controls on these risk scores about 80% of the time. We proposed a final seven-point risk assessment instrument that might be tested to identify potential homicide offenders in childhood.

We conclude that homicide offending can be predicted surprisingly well in childhood but that there are many false positives. We will try to overcome this false-positive problem in Chap. 5.

Chapter 5
Prediction of Homicide Offenders Out of Violent Boys

David P. Farrington and Rolf Loeber

In Chap. 4, we investigated the extent to which convicted homicide offenders could be predicted from factors measured in childhood in a population of youth from public schools. One of the problems with predicting homicide offenders out of the whole population is that the false-positive errors can be high, because many individuals who are predicted to offend who do not in fact offend (Loeber et al., 2005a). For example, in Chap. 4, we concluded that about 8–14% of high-risk boys became convicted homicide offenders, giving a false-positive rate of 86–92%.

A strategy to improve the prediction of rare phenomena is to undertake stepwise prediction (Loeber et al., 2005a). Stepwise prediction involves three steps: (a) first determine which factor is a common antecedent among homicide offenders; (b) identify predictors of the common antecedent, and (c) predict homicide among those who possess the common antecedent. Stepwise prediction has the advantage of increasing the base-rate of homicide in the subpopulation who share the common antecedent, and hence of decreasing the false-positive rate. The other advantage is that this strategy allows us to explore the question of whether predictors of homicide offenders are qualitatively different from predictors of violent individuals. In other words, are there predictors of homicide offenders that are unique and that are not predictors of violent individuals?

Earlier analyses (Loeber et al., 2005a) established that a common factor among most of the convicted homicide offenders was that they had been violent (based either on self-reports or convictions for aggravated assault or robbery) before committing the murder. This was true of 35 of the 37 homicide offenders (95%) in the present study. Thus, we can categorically state that, in most instances of homicide committed by young men in the PYS, the homicide appears at a later point of a life in which the commission of violence appears at an earlier stage of development. The earlier analyses (Loeber et al., 2005a) proceeded by first predicting violence among the whole population of youth and, after that, by predicting homicide among those who had been violent.

We are also interested in the extent to which predictors of homicide offending overlap with predictors of violence (other than homicide). We are particularly

R. Loeber and D.P. Farrington, *Young Homicide Offenders and Victims*,
Longitudinal Research in the Social and Behavioral Sciences: An Interdisciplinary Series,
DOI 10.1007/978-1-4419-9949-8_5, © Springer Science+Business Media, LLC 2011

keen to know to what extent predictors of homicide offending are quantitatively or qualitatively different from predictors of violence. In the earlier analyses (Loeber et al., 2005a), we found more evidence for quantitative rather than qualitative differences. In general, risk factors for homicide offending were similar to risk factors for violence, but the homicide offenders were more extreme, in having more risk factors.

Another important question is the degree to which there is a dose–response relationship between the number of risk factors predicting violence and the probability of later violence. Earlier analyses (Loeber et al., 2005a; Loeber & Pardini, 2008) showed a steady increase in the likelihood of later violence as the number of risk factors increased. Similarly, we wanted to examine whether a dose–response relationship exists between the number of risk factors and the probability of later homicide offending.

Another issue is whether predictors of homicide offending recorded early in life add to predictive efficiency even when later predictors measured in adolescence are taken into account. Along one train of thought, it can be argued that predictors measured during adolescence, being more proximal to homicide offending, might overshadow earlier predictors measured during childhood. However, another possibility is that predictors of homicide offending involve an accumulation of disadvantages (measured by risk factors) of which some occur early in life and others occur later, especially among future homicide offenders. In the latter case, we would find that significant predictors of homicide offending measured in childhood had independent predictive contributions alongside risk factors measured during adolescence.

The present analyses differ from the earlier published analyses (Loeber et al., 2005a) in that: (1) they are based on a larger sample of homicide offenders (37 compared to 33); (2) they use odds ratios rather than chi-squared to measure predictive efficiency; (3) they use logistic regression rather than the Burgess method to develop a risk score; and (4) they use unweighted data so that individuals can be studied. The use of weighted data and the listwise elimination of missing cases in the Loeber et al. (2005a) paper meant that the risk score analyses of the predictors of homicide offenders were based on very small numbers (only 23 homicide offenders in Table 5 of that paper). In the analyses that follow, we use unweighted data and pro-rate risk scores so that all 37 homicide offenders are included in our risk score analyses.

The analyses are based on the 37 convicted homicide offenders and two comparison groups: 652 violent boys (according to self-reports or official records of index violence) who did not commit homicide and 754 nonviolent boys. Of the remaining 74 boys in the PYS, four died and one emigrated permanently by age 14, 33 were arrested for homicide but not convicted, and 36 were homicide victims. (Of the other three homicide victims, two were convicted homicide offenders, and one was an arrested homicide offender.)

The prevalence of violent boys in the PYS was very high. Only seven of the homicide victims were not violent, totalling 761 nonviolent boys. Excluding the 5 not known boys, the remaining 751 were violent (including violent boys and convicted and arrested homicide offenders). Therefore, the prevalence of violence was 49.7% (61.4% of African Americans vs. 34.2% of Caucasians; OR=3.1, CI=2.5–3.8).

Weighting back to the Pittsburgh Public School population, the prevalence of violence was 44.2% (55.8% of African Americans vs. 29.4% of Caucasians; OR = 3.0, CI = 2.4–3.8).

In summary, this chapter addresses the following questions:

- Is the prediction of homicide offenders more efficient when based on those who were violent earlier in life compared to a prediction based on the general population of youth?
- Are predictors of homicide offenders qualitatively different from predictors of violent individuals?
- Do predictors recorded in childhood continue to predict convicted homicide offenders even when predictors recorded in adolescence are taken into account?

In the final section of this chapter, we combine the convicted and arrested homicide offenders. Some of the arrested (but not convicted) offenders indeed committed murder, but others did not. Therefore, analyses only of the convicted homicide offenders underestimate the true prevalence of homicide offending, and possibly focus on a biased sample of homicide offenders. In contrast, analyses of the convicted plus arrested offenders overestimates prevalence but possibly gives a more accurate indication of the false-positive rate and might go some way toward correcting the bias and revealing the true characteristics of homicide offenders. These analyses have to be tentative because we cannot be certain about how many of the arrested but not convicted boys were truly guilty.

Predicting Violent Boys

We started with the 63 risk factors used by Loeber et al. (2005a) in their analyses, several of which were based on multiple waves of data (see Chap. 2). To expand the range of possible risk factors, we added 14 factors studied in Chap. 4 (measured in childhood, at the beginning of the study) that were not included in those earlier analyses. Seven were behavioral factors which usually are correlated with and/or precursors to violence, including serious delinquency, nonphysical aggression, runs away, positive attitude to delinquency, bad relationship with peers, suspended, and negative attitude to school. We also included seven explanatory factors (i.e., not directly related to the boy's deviant behavior) including lack of guilt, HIA (hyperactivity, impulsivity, and attention problems), low achievement (according to the California Achievement Test), broken home, large family size, a small house, and an unemployed mother. All these factors were measured in the screening and first follow-up assessments in 1987–1988, when the boys were aged 7–13.

Of these 77 candidate predictors, 17 risk factors were deleted for the following reasons: 11 did not predict violent boys or homicide offenders (low birth weight, perinatal problems, developmental delays, parent help-seeking for the boy's depression or alcohol/drug problems or learning problems, unconventional peers, poorly educated mother, parents disagree on discipline, discipline not persistent, and positive attitude to problem behavior). The diagnoses of ADHD, CD, and ODD were also deleted because they were all subsumed under disruptive behavior disorder. Two or more caretaker changes before age 10 was deleted because the construct had more missing data than the broken family construct. Delinquency onset before age 10 was deleted because it overlapped with the more important serious delinquency variable. Parental help-seeking for child behavior problems/ truancy was deleted because it overlapped with the more important truancy measure used in Chap. 4. This left 59 risk factors, of which 29 were explanatory and 30 were behavioral, plus race ethnicity. Thus, in this chapter, because of the emphasis on prediction from childhood *and* adolescence, a wider range of risk factors (59) is studied here than in Chap. 4 (where we studied 40 risk factors) which focused on predictive factors measured in childhood only.

As suggested by prior research, there were racial/ethnic differences in the prevalence of violent boys and convicted homicide offenders. Of the 652 violent boys, 439 (67%) were African American, compared with 326 (43%) of the 754 nonviolent boys (OR=2.7, CI=2.2–3.4). Of the 37 convicted homicide offenders, 32 (86%) were African American, compared with 439 (67%) of the 652 violent boys (OR=2.1, CI=1.2–8.1). These odds ratios for race are not particularly high and are lower than the corresponding odds ratios for many other risk factors.

How well do risk factors measured during childhood and adolescence predict violence? Table 5.1 shows that 58 out of the 59 factors predicted violent boys. One factor (a positive attitude to substance use) did not significantly predict violent boys (but, as will be shown later, a positive attitude to substance use significantly predicted convicted homicide offenders). Risk factors from all domains significantly contributed to the prediction of violence (including explanatory factors in the child and parent, child-rearing practices, birth measures, socioeconomic factors; and also behavioral factors, including child variables, child attitude, parent, peer, school, and delinquency). For example, 9% of the mothers of nonviolent boys used alcohol during pregnancy, compared to 15% of the mothers of violent boys (OR=1.6), and the respective figures for recorded child abuse were 9% and 23% (OR=2.9). Among the explanatory factors, the strongest predictors of violent boys were callous-unemotional behavior (OR=6.0) and lack of guilt (OR=4.2), followed by HIA (OR=3.2) and broken home (OR=3.1). Among the behavioral factors, the strongest predictors were prior serious delinquency (OR=9.8), which is not surprising, sold hard drugs (OR=9.3), sold marijuana (OR=8.1), gun carrying (OR=6.9), nonphysical aggression (OR=6.8), and gang fighting (OR=5.0). None of the nonviolent males used a weapon.

It should be pointed out that (unlike the analyses of homicide offenders) these analyses are not strictly predictive. In some cases, the violence could have occurred before the risk factor. Nevertheless, the term "prediction" is used here, for convenience. All of the risk factors were measured before anyone was convicted for homicide.

Violence Risk Score. Which predictors measured during childhood and adolescence best predicted violent boys? Table 5.2 shows the results of a logistic regression analysis to establish the independent predictors of violent compared with nonviolent boys. Most of the best predictors were earlier measures of antisocial behavior

Table 5.1 Predicting violent boys and convicted homicide offenders

Risk factor	Percent of			Odds ratio	
	Nonviolent boys (754)	Violent boys (652)	Homicide offenders (37)	V-NV	H-V
Explanatory factors					
Birth (3)					
Prenatal problems	30	37	38	1.4*	1.0
Mother cigarette use	42	49	55	1.3*	1.3
Mother alcohol use	9	15	13	1.6*	0.8
Child behaviors (9)					
Lack of guilt	13	38	43	4.2*	1.3
Callous-unemotional	10	40	35	6.0*	0.8
HIA	10	26	30	3.2*	1.2
Old for the grade	19	32	49	2.0*	2.1*
Low achievement (CAT)	16	33	29	2.5*	0.8
Low achievement (PT)	17	32	30	2.3*	0.9
Depressed mood	17	30	30	2.2*	1.0
Shy/withdrawn	22	33	38	1.8*	1.2
Boy not involved	20	29	27	1.6*	0.9
Family functioning (6)					
Young mother	16	27	45	1.9*	2.2*
Broken home	18	25	24	1.5*	0.9
Father behavior problems	12	23	32	2.2*	1.6
Parent substance use	21	35	32	2.0*	0.9
Parent stress	20	33	30	2.0*	0.9
Police contact relatives	35	45	52	1.6*	1.3
Child rearing (4)					
Poor supervision	21	33	30	1.8*	0.9
Physical punishment	20	30	32	1.7*	1.1
Poor communication	18	35	35	2.4*	1.0
Child abuse	9	23	27	2.9*	1.3
Family socioeconomic (5)					
Low SES	19	34	43	2.2*	1.5
Family on welfare	33	54	71	2.4*	2.0
Large family size	50	76	89	3.1*	2.6
Small house	19	31	31	1.9*	1.0
Unemployed mother	22	27	45	1.3*	2.2*
Neighborhood (2)					
Bad neighborhood (C)	22	43	65	2.7*	2.4*
Bad neighborhood (P)	18	32	30	2.2*	0.9
Behavioral factors					
Child (9)					
Serious delinquency	10	51	57	9.8*	1.3
Covert behavior	12	39	46	4.7*	1.4
Physical aggression	12	42	30	5.3*	0.6
Nonphysical aggression	10	43	38	6.8*	0.8
Cruel to people	9	42	43	7.5*	1.0
Cruel to animals	8	14	16	1.8*	1.2

(continued)

Table 5.1 (continued)

Risk factor	Percent of			Odds ratio	
	Nonviolent boys (754)	Violent boys (652)	Homicide offenders (37)	V-NV	H-V
Runs away	12	20	24	1.9*	1.3
Disruptive behavior disorder	15	32	51	2.7*	2.2*
High-risk score	33	67	81	4.1*	2.1
Child attitude (3)					
Positive attitude to delinquency	19	28	54	1.7*	3.0*
Positive attitude to substance use	22	26	46	1.2	2.4*
Unlikely to get caught	20	31	22	1.8*	0.6
Parent (2)					
Bad relationship with parent	17	32	32	2.3*	1.0
Counter control	23	34	27	1.8*	0.7
Peer (4)					
Peer delinquency	16	33	49	2.5*	1.9*
Peer substance use	11	20	36	2.1*	2.3*
Bad friends	19	32	41	2.0*	1.5
Bad relationship with peers	13	40	35	4.4*	0.8
School (4)					
Suspended	28	60	78	3.8*	2.4*
Truant	27	50	54	2.7*	1.2
Negative attitude to school	24	32	19	1.5*	0.5
Low school motivation	23	53	51	3.9*	0.9
Offending (8)					
Weapon carrying	7	17	41	2.8*	3.4*
Gun carrying	2	11	18	6.9*	1.8
Weapon use	0	17	25	X	1.6
Gang membership	6	23	29	4.8*	1.4
Gang fighting	2	9	22	5.0*	2.8*
Persistent drug use	13	25	38	2.1*	1.8
Sold marijuana	2	15	25	8.1*	1.8
Sold hard drugs	2	14	28	9.3*	2.3*

Notes: *$p < .05$; X OR = 139.7 if the zero cell is replaced by 1. V-NV concerns the comparison between violent boys and nonviolent boys; H-V concerns the comparison between homicide offenders and violent boys. *P* parent, *T* teacher, *C* census, *CAT* California Achievement Test, *HIA* hyperactivity–impulsivity–attention deficit. Weapon carrying and gang fighting in this table are different from the constructs with the same names in Chap. 4. The variables in this table were measured at wave E (see Table 2.3). The variables in Chap. 4 were cumulative measures up to age 14

Table 5.2 Multiple regression analyses to predict violent boys

Risk factor	LRCS change	p	Partial OR	p
Serious delinquency	265.90	.0001	5.6	.0001
Cruel to people	75.38	.0001	3.0	.0001
Gang member	48.16	.0001	2.7	.0004
Bad neighborhood (C)	29.02	.0001	2.1	.0001
Callous-unemotional	23.98	.0001	2.1	.001
Poor communication	12.41	.0004	1.8	.002
Sold marijuana	11.91	.0006	2.3	.036
Suspended	9.72	.002	1.6	.006
Low school motivation	5.50	.019	1.5	.027
Sold hard drugs	5.68	.017	2.9	.026
Gun carrying	4.12	.042	2.5	.045
Broken family	2.89	.089	1.3	.089
African American	9.92	.003	1.9	.002

Notes: LRCS likelihood ratio chi-squared, *OR* odds ratio, *(C)* census

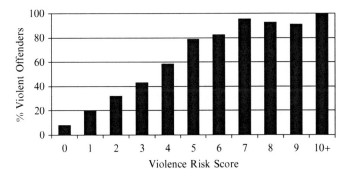

Fig. 5.1 Violence risk score predicting violent boys

(serious delinquency, cruel to people, gang membership, sold marijuana, suspended from school, sold hard drugs, and gun carrying). The most important explanatory predictors were callous-unemotional behavior, living in a bad neighborhood, poor parent–boy communication, and coming from a broken home. After controlling for all 12 predictors, African American race still predicted violent boys.

Next, we examined the extent to which there is a dose–response relationship between the number of risk factors and the probability of later violence. To answer this question, a violence risk score was calculated based on the number of risk factors out of 12. Figure 5.1 shows a clear dose–response relationship: The higher the number of risk factors, the higher the probability of becoming a violent boy. The percentage of violent boys increased from 8% of those with no risk factors to 100% of those with ten or more risk factors. Note that the maximum predictability was almost achieved at seven risk factors. The area under the ROC curve (AUC) was .832 (SD = .011). Of 249 boys scoring six or more, 90% were violent, compared with 37% of 1,154 scoring five or less (OR = 16.0, CI = 10.3–24.8). Of 390 boys scoring five or more, 86% were violent, compared with 31% of 1,013 scoring four or less (OR = 13.8, CI = 10.0–18.9). In summary, the results show a generally increasing dose–response relationship between the number of risk factors and the probability of later violence. The spread of the risk score is from 8 to 100%, which compared to other studies is amazingly high. For example, in predicting violence in the Cambridge Study, only about half of the high-risk group became violent (Farrington, 2001a). However, as mentioned, the present analyses are not strictly predictive.

The predictors of violent boys documented in these analyses largely replicate those found in other studies (e.g., Farrington, 1998; Hawkins, Laub, & Lauritsen, 1998; Lipsey & Derzon, 1998), and not surprisingly overlap with those reported by Loeber et al. (2005a) for the smaller sample of homicide offenders in PYS. However, the present results show that several factors not included in the earlier analyses predicted violence, including lack of guilt, HIA, low achievement (CAT), broken home, large family size, a small house, and an unemployed mother. Of these extra variables, only a broken home contributed independently (but weakly) in the logistic regression predicting violent boys. The other risk factors which independently contributed to the prediction were mostly behavioral; among the strongest were prior serious delinquency, selling hard drugs, gun carrying, cruelty to people, and gang membership. None of these factors will come as a surprise to experts in violence, and they largely serve to confirm that the results based on the PYS are in line with other major findings (see Loeber & Farrington, 1998).

The results may seem to lend strong support for the screening of individuals at risk of violence, but caution is warranted. A cutoff point of six or more risk factors produced an OR of 16.0, whereas a cutoff point of five or more risk factors produced an OR of 13.8. These ORs are substantially higher than those reported in the earlier analyses (Loeber et al., 2005a) when a cutoff point of four or more was used (OR = 6.0). In the present analyses, a cutoff point of five or more produced a high false-negative rate (31%), and a lower false-positive rate (14%), with a sensitivity of 52% (336 out of 651) and a specificity of 93% (698 out of 752). The positive predictive power (the proportion of individuals identified as likely violent boys who became violent boys) was 86% (336 out of 390), while the negative predictive power (the proportion of individuals identified as nonviolent boys who actually became nonviolent boys) was 69% (698 out of 1,013). The fact that so many violent boys (48%) were missed in this prediction exercise is worrisome to us, and does not provide a strong backing for the use of the results for screening purposes (especially since predictive accuracy is over-estimated here).

Predicting Convicted Homicide Offenders Out of Violent Boys

Is the prediction of homicide offenders more efficient when based on those who were violent earlier in life compared to a prediction based on the general population of youth? For the following analyses, we will compare the 37 homicide offenders with the other 652 violent boys. The right-hand column of Table 5.1 shows that four

Table 5.3 Independent predictors of convicted homicide offenders

Risk factor	LRCS change	p	Partial OR	p
Weapon carrying	8.90	.003	3.5	.003
Bad neighborhood (C)	8.31	.004	2.5	.031
Young mother	5.06	.025	2.5	.021
Positive attitude to substance use	3.88	.049	2.2	.050
Suspended	3.93	.047	2.7	.056
Unemployed mother	3.15	.076	2.0	.073

Notes: LRCS likelihood ratio chi-squared, *OR* odds ratio, *(C)* census

explanatory factors significantly discriminated between homicide offenders and other violent boys: old for the grade (held back), a young mother, an unemployed mother, and a bad neighborhood according to census data. A broken home had a high OR (2.6) but this was not significant because of the high prevalence of broken families among both violent boys (76%) and homicide offenders (89%).

Table 5.1 also shows that nine behavioral factors significantly predicted convicted homicide offenders among violent boys, including disruptive behavior disorder, a positive attitude toward delinquency, a positive attitude toward substance use, peer delinquency, peer substance use, weapon carrying, gang fighting, and sold hard drugs. Thus, in total, 13 out of the 59 risk factors (22%) significantly predicted homicide offenders, which was much greater than the 5% expected by chance alone. In particular, homicide offenders were more than twice as likely as other violent boys to carry a weapon (41% compared with 17%; OR = 3.4), to sell hard drugs (28% compared with 14%; OR = 2.3), and to be involved in gang fighting (22% compared with 9%; OR = 2.8).

The results show that, with only one exception, the predictors of homicide offending were a subset of the predictors of violence. In other words, numerous risk factors were characteristic of violent boys, and some of these were even more characteristic of homicide offenders, indicating that they differed in degree but not in kind from violent boys. The one exception was the factor of a positive attitude to substance use. Violent and nonviolent boys did not differ significantly on this factor, but more of the homicide offenders had a positive attitude to substance use than did the violent boys (46% vs. 26%; OR = 2.4). However, in light of the fact that the related variable of a positive attitude to delinquency predicted both violent boys and homicide offenders, we do not conclude that this single result is evidence of a difference in kind between violent boys and homicide offenders.

Logistic regression analyses were carried out to investigate the independent predictors of convicted homicide offenders out of all violent boys. Table 5.3 shows that six factors contributed to the prediction of homicide offenders: weapon carrying, a bad neighborhood according to the census, a young mother, a positive attitude to substance use, suspended from school, and an unemployed mother. Thus, two sets of factors were pivotal in the prediction of homicide offenders out of the violent boys: indicators of the mother's disadvantage and indicators of the youth's problem behavior, both passive (attitude to substance use) and proactive (weapon carrying).

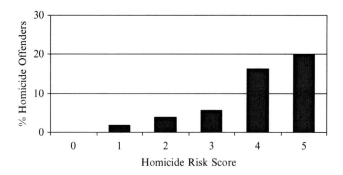

Fig. 5.2 Risk score predicting convicted homicide offenders out of violent boys

After controlling for all six significant or near-significant predictors, race did not predict convicted homicide offenders. Thus, although most homicide offenders were of African American race, their race did not contribute to the prediction of those who would eventually kill or not, after controlling for other risk factors.

Homicide Risk Score. We constructed a homicide risk score predicting homicide offenders among violent boys on the basis of the six factors identified in the logistic regression analyses. This homicide risk score was based on the number of risk factors out of 6. Figure 5.2 shows a steadily increasing dose–response function: the percentage who committed homicide increased from 0% of those with no risk factors to 20% of those with five risk factors. (No boy had all six risk factors.) In these analyses, the AUC was .763 (SD = .038), which indicated a moderately strong predictive relationship; in 76% of cases, homicide offenders had higher scores than violent boys.

The most remarkable result is that the percentage of convicted homicide offenders among high-risk violent boys (20%) was hardly greater than the percentage of convicted homicide offenders among boys in the total sample with high behavioral risk scores (17%; see Chap. 4). Also, the AUC in the present analysis (.763) is very similar to the AUC in that previous analysis (.773; Fig. 4.2). Therefore, predicting homicide offenders out of violent boys, and including risk factors measured after the beginning of the study in 1987–1988, did not significantly improve predictive accuracy. It may be that the predictive accuracy found in Chap. 4, and the percentage of high-risk boys who are convicted for homicide, is close to the maximum possible, given the unpredictability of homicide convictions.

Based on the results of the ROC analyses, the homicide risk score was dichotomized to identify the 15% at highest risk, with four or five of the risk factors. Nearly half (18 out of 37, or 49%) of the homicide offenders were among the high-risk boys. This produced an OR of 6.1 (CI = 3.1–12.0). A cutoff point of three or higher produced an OR of 4.6 (CI = 2.2–9.5). Because the false negatives are lower with a cutoff point of three or more (see below), this is the cutoff point that we considered to be the most optimal. Those violent boys who scored three or more on the homicide prediction scale were four times as likely to commit homicide compared to those who scored two or less (10.5% compared with 2.5%).

In this comparison, the sensitivity (the proportion of homicide offenders who were correctly classified as homicide offenders) was 70% (26 out of 37), while the specificity (the proportion of nonhomicide offenders correctly classified as nonhomicide offenders) was 66% (429 out of 650). The positive predictive power (the proportion of individuals identified as likely homicide offenders who became homicide offenders) was 11% (26 out of 247), while the negative predictive power (the proportion of individuals identified as nonhomicide offenders who were nonhomicide offenders) was 98% (429 out of 440). The proportion of false-negative errors (the proportion of homicide offenders classified as nonhomicide offenders) was 30% (11 out of 37), while the proportion of false-positive errors (the proportion of individuals classified as likely homicide offenders who were not homicide offenders) was 89% (221 out of 247). This is still a very high false-positive rate.

Another question addressed in this chapter is whether predictors recorded in childhood continue to predict convicted homicide offenders even when predictors recorded in adolescence are taken into account. In the logistic regression analysis (Table 5.3), three explanatory factors measured during childhood, namely a bad neighborhood, a young mother, and an unemployed mother, continued to predict homicide offending even when behavioral and later more proximal factors were taken into account (i.e., weapon carrying, suspended from school, and a positive attitude to substance use). Thus, the results indicate that early family handicaps such as a bad neighborhood, a young mother, and unemployment of the mother may constitute a platform of risk from which other risk factors may flow, particularly uncontrolled juvenile behaviors such as a positive attitude to substance use and problem behavior leading to school suspension, which in turn are likely to increase the probability of carrying a weapon and the commission of homicide later.

Estimation of True Prediction

Because the homicide risk score in Fig. 5.2 was calculated in light of knowledge about which risk factors were the best predictors of convicted homicide offenders, predictive accuracy is over-estimated. In order to derive more accurate estimates of predictive accuracy, the screening risk score (measured at ages 7–13) and the number of arrests up to age 14 were studied. Figure 5.3 shows the extent to which the screening risk score predicted homicide offenders out of all violent boys. There was only a weak dose–response relationship, and the predictive efficiency was disappointing at AUC = .587 (n.s.; SD = .049). This prediction was much poorer than the prediction of homicide offenders out of the whole population (AUC = .709, Fig. 4.3) and the odds ratios were also lower: OR = 2.0 (CI = 1.0–3.9) for a cutoff of five or more risk factors, and OR = 1.7 (CI = 0.8–3.7) for a cutoff of six or more risk factors. The false-positive rate was hardly improved (91% here for the highest scores, compared with 92% based on Fig. 4.3).

As a second test, Fig. 5.4 shows the extent to which the number of arrests up to age 14 predicted homicide offenders out of all violent boys. The predictability here is much better than with the screening risk score. Of the 83 violent boys with nine

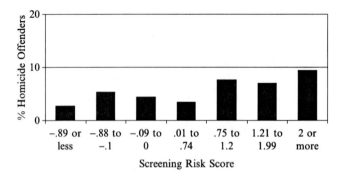

Fig. 5.3 Screening risk score predicting convicted homicide offenders out of violent boys

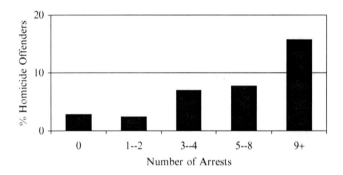

Fig. 5.4 Arrests up to age 14 predicting convicted homicide offenders out of the violent boys

or more arrests, 15% became homicide offenders, comprising 35% of all homicide offenders. Of the 160 violent boys with five or more arrests, 12% became homicide offenders, comprising 51% of all homicide offenders. For the number of arrests, AUC = .698 (SD = .054), but this is still less than the comparable AUC for predicting homicide offenders out of the whole population (AUC = .794, which we reported in Chap. 4). The odds ratios were also lower here: OR = 4.5 (CI = 2.2–9.2) for a cutoff of nine or more risk factors; OR = 3.8 (CI = 2.0–7.5) for a cutoff of five or more risk factors. It clearly seems harder to predict homicide offenders out of violent boys than out of the whole population. The false-positive rate was slightly improved in Fig. 5.4 [84% for those with nine or more arrests, compared with 87% (Chap. 4)].

Predicting Convicted Plus Arrested Homicide Offenders

As mentioned earlier, when the 33 boys arrested (but not convicted) for homicide are added to the 37 convicted homicide offenders, the resulting category of 70 boys may possibly constitute a less biased sample of homicide offenders, although some

Table 5.4 Independent predictors of arrested/convicted homicide offenders

Risk factor	LRCS change	p	Partial OR	p
Gang fighting	12.64	.0004	2.7	.006
Truant	7.00	.008	2.0	.030
Young mother	5.53	.019	2.0	.022
Peer substance use	4.83	.028	1.9	.048
Positive attitude to delinquency	3.01	.083	1.7	.079
African American	13.69	.0002	4.6	.002

Notes: *LRCS* likelihood ratio chi-squared, *OR* odds ratio

of the arrested boys are not guilty. Eleven of the risk factors listed in Table 5.1 significantly predicted the combined homicide offenders out of the violent boys: gang fighting (OR = 3.0), a broken home (OR = 2.1), peer substance use (OR = 2.1), old for the grade (OR = 2.0), peer delinquency (OR = 2.0), a positive attitude to delinquency (OR = 2.0), weapon carrying (OR = 2.0), truancy (OR = 1.9), suspended from school (OR = 1.9), disruptive behavior disorder (OR = 1.8), and a young mother (OR = 1.8).

Nine of these 11 risk factors also significantly predicted convicted homicide offenders: all except a broken home (which had a large OR = 2.6 in Table 5.1) and truancy (OR = 1.2). Conversely, 9 of the 13 risk factors that significantly predicted convicted homicide offenders also significantly predicted the combined offenders: all except a positive attitude to substance use (which was very nearly significant: OR = 1.7, CI = 0.98–2.8), an unemployed mother, a bad neighborhood according to the census, and selling hard drugs. Not surprisingly, therefore, the best predictors of convicted homicide offenders (out of the violent boys) were generally similar to the best predictors of the combined group of homicide offenders.

Table 5.4 shows that the independently important predictors of convicted plus arrested homicide offenders were gang fighting, truancy, a young mother, peer substance use, and a positive attitude to delinquency. Only one of these five factors (a young mother) was also an independent predictor of convicted homicide offenders in the general population (see Table 4.8). After controlling for these five factors, African American race was still a significant predictor of combined homicide offenders, which was not the case for the prediction of convicted homicide offenders. As pointed out in Chap. 4, race was more strongly related to homicide arrestees (OR = 13.0) than to convicted homicide offenders (OR = 5.4), possibly because there is more bias involved in an arrest than in a conviction.

Arrested/Convicted Homicide Score. A risk score was then calculated based on the five independent predictors of combined homicide offenders. Figure 5.5 shows that the percentage of boys who became combined homicide offenders increased from 4% of boys with no risk factors to 29% of boys with four or five risk factors. Compared with the prediction of convicted homicide offenders, the false-positive rate was lower in this analysis (71% compared with 80% in Fig. 5.2). However, the predictive accuracy was much lower for combined homicide offenders (AUC = .649) than for convicted homicide offenders (AUC = .763; SD = .037). It seems likely that

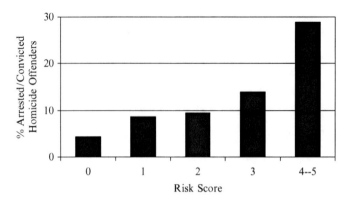

Fig. 5.5 Risk score predicting arrested/convicted homicide offenders out of violent boys

the combined homicide offenders are harder to predict because they include some boys who are not in fact homicide offenders. Therefore, the advantages of including more presumed homicide offenders seem to be outweighed by the disadvantages of including nonhomicide offenders.

Conclusions

This chapter advances the field of homicide studies in several ways. First, it reports on young male homicide offenders and other violent boys who were studied for many years prior to when the homicide and the violence were committed. The reports of violence were based on information from multiple sources (youth, parent, teacher, and official delinquency records), while homicide offending was based on conviction as a result of a trial in court. Second, a large variety of risk factors in multiple domains was studied, based on multiple sources of information. The study highlights the great variety of predictors, some occurring early in life, which can be used in forecasting violence, which may reflect the multicausal nature of violence.

The analyses in this chapter have several limitations. The classification of self-reported violent or nonviolent offending was based on all available data up to wave 18 (2001) for the youngest cohort, wave 14 (1998) for the oldest cohort, but only up to wave 7 (1991) for the middle cohort. Therefore, the data would not reflect later changes in the middle cohort's self-reported offending. The earliest measurement of risk factors was at age 7 for the youngest cohort, age 10 for the middle cohort, and at age 13 for the oldest cohort. The number of prospective assessments of the middle cohort was limited to 7 waves and did not go beyond age 13, which meant that the assessment of risk factors was before the homicide offending (although not always before the violence).

Our results show that it is possible to predict violence, and that the prediction is actually stronger than in the earlier analyses with a slightly smaller number of homicide offenders (Loeber et al., 2005a). The univariate results show that a wide range of explanatory and behavioral factors contributed to the prediction, many of which are also known from other longitudinal studies (e.g., Farrington, 2007b). Among the explanatory variables were factors situated in the child, the parent, child-rearing practices, birth-related problems, and socioeconomic factors. Many of the explanatory and behavioral factors are potentially malleable and could be targeted on as part of preventive interventions, a point to which we will return in the final chapter of this volume.

We also found that it is possible to predict homicide offenders out of the population of young violent males. The predictors included both long-term risk factors (e.g., a young mother, an unemployed mother, suspended from school) and more proximal risk factors, such as weapon carrying. However, predictive analyses based on a homicide risk score had a high rate of false-positive errors (80%) showing that a high proportion of youth with five risk factors did not commit homicide, at least judging from the available criminal history record information. However, all of the individuals in this false-positive group were not "innocent" individuals but were known for their violence.

Disappointingly but also interestingly, predicting convicted homicide offenders out of the violent boys, and adding later risk factors, did not increase predictive accuracy and did not reduce the false-positive rate very much. Comparing the prediction of convicted homicide offenders out of violent boys with the prediction of convicted homicide offenders out of the whole sample, the false-positive rate decreased only from 83 to 80%, and the AUCs were virtually identical. In comparable genuine prediction exercises using the screening risk score and the number of arrests up to age 14, predictive accuracy was lower in predicting convicted homicide offenders out of violent boys compared with out of the total population, and the false-positive rates were not reduced by much. It may truly be harder to predict homicide offenders out of a more homogeneous group of violent boys than out of the whole sample.

Generally, the predictors of homicide offending were similar to the predictors of violence, suggesting that homicide offenders differ in degree but not in kind from violent boys. Even after including later risk factors, early explanatory factors were still important in these predictions, including being old for the grade (held back), a young mother, an unemployed mother, and a bad neighborhood. Early behavioral factors were also important, including a diagnosis of disruptive behavior disorder, positive attitudes to delinquency and substance use, peer delinquency, peer substance use, and suspended from school. There was a dose–response relationship between the number of risk factors and the likelihood of becoming a convicted homicide offender.

The finding that half of the homicide offenders received a research diagnosis of disruptive behavior disorder should be interpreted with caution. Many of the symptoms of disruptive behavior disorder are acting out behaviors and, therefore, may only reflect the continuity of antisocial behaviors over time, albeit with an escalation in severity culminating in murder. We stress that the findings do not mean that all children who qualify for a diagnosis of disruptive behavior disorder are at risk of becoming homicide offenders. Nevertheless, the data presented show that such a diagnosis early in life, when accompanied by other risk factors, increased the risk of homicide offending among violent boys.

The role of African American race in the prediction exercises is still somewhat perplexing. We found that most violence and homicide in the PYS was committed by African American young men (see also Loeber et al., 2005a; Loeber, Farrington, Stouthamer-Loeber, & White, 2008). However, whereas those earlier analyses did not find that African American race predicted violence once other risk factors were known, in the present analyses African American status remained significant in the logistic regression predicting violence even after entering other significant risk factors. On the other hand, in the prediction of convicted homicide offenders, African American race did not contribute to the equation. The results are not relevant for possible interventions because African American race does not fall into the category of risk factors that can be reduced by intervention. However, assuming that African American boys are more at risk because they have more early risk factors, these early risk factors could be targeted in intervention programs.

The findings on modifiable risk factors have implications for the prevention of homicide offending. Specifically, reducing risk factors that are significantly associated with homicide may help reduce homicide offending. Situational crime prevention strategies, such as preventing youth from carrying weapons, affiliating with delinquent peers, participating in gang fights, and/or selling drugs are important. These observations may have an "oh, we already know this" ring because these risk factors often are incorporated into gang reduction programs (Howell, 1998). At the same time, the findings in the present study indicate that long-term risk factors need to be tackled as well, including nondelinquent antisocial behavior (Loeber & Farrington, 2001), and also attitudes that favor or facilitate antisocial behaviors. We will revisit the issue of prevention and intervention in Chaps. 8 and 9, which demonstrate new nonexperimental ways to model the impact of interventions on later violence and homicide offending.

Chapter 6
Early Risk Factors for Homicide Victims and Shooting Victims

David P. Farrington and Rolf Loeber

It is well known that homicide offenders and their victims have many characteristics in common (Broidy et al., 2003; Federal Bureau of Investigation, 2003; Snyder & Sickmund, 1999). Less clear is the extent to which predictors of homicide offenders are similar to the predictors of homicide victims. The reason is the scarcity of longitudinal studies which have information from diverse informants about the early antecedents of homicide victimization. Two major sets of questions are important here.

- How common are homicide victims in Pittsburgh?
- To what extent did homicide victims engage in antisocial and delinquent behaviors before they were killed?
- Which explanatory, behavioral, and criminal risk factors predict homicide victims out of a community sample up to 22 years later?
- Is there a dose–response relationship between the number of risk factors and the probability of becoming a homicide victim?
- To what extent can homicide victims be predicted based on a combination of explanatory, behavioral, and criminal risk factors?

In a second set of questions, we want to compare homicide victims and homicide offenders, and address the following questions:

- Are homicide offenders and victims similar in their antisocial behavior?
- Did homicide offenders, compared to homicide victims, grow up under more deprived conditions or were they exposed to more risk factors?
- Do early risk factors predict homicide offenders more accurately than homicide victims?

We also address the following key questions pertaining to shooting victims who did not die:

- Which explanatory, behavioral, and criminal risk factors predict shooting victims?
- How accurately can shooting victims be predicted?

R. Loeber and D.P. Farrington, *Young Homicide Offenders and Victims*,
Longitudinal Research in the Social and Behavioral Sciences: An Interdisciplinary Series,
DOI 10.1007/978-1-4419-9949-8_6, © Springer Science+Business Media, LLC 2011

- Is there a dose–response relationship between the number of risk factors and the probability of becoming a shooting victim?
- To what extent are the predictors of shooting victims similar to the predictors of homicide victims?
- Are racial differences in the prevalence of homicide and shooting victims attributable to racial differences in early risk factors?

Given that there are many shared characteristics between violent offenders and victims of violence, there are several possible explanations for the overlap. In a simple conceptualization, violence begets violence, and the victims of violence result from a reciprocal process of violent interactions. Since most homicides involve shooting, perhaps homicide offenders shoot more quickly or more accurately than homicide victims. Second, violence may not necessarily be the result of a reciprocal process of aggression, but more the result of a selection effect in which individuals with aggressive predispositions meet each other and become embroiled in violence. Popular theories suggest that offenders and victims have similar lifestyles and routine activities, and live in similar disadvantaged, disorganized neighborhoods. Yet a third possibility is that violence evolves from other disputes related to illegal activities, such as the drug trade, the trade in stolen goods, robbery to obtain drugs and/or money, or other illegal property transactions. The following analyses can address these different possible causes and can shed light on which activities put individuals at risk of becoming a victim of shooting and/or homicide.

The analyses will also shed light on childhood predictors of homicide victims and shooting victims, and on the extent to which convicted homicide offenders and homicide victims were exposed to similar sets of risk factors in their childhood. For instance, are similar family factors implicated in the prediction of homicide offenders as well as homicide victims? And is the same true for other social conditions of neighborhood deprivation? It is also important to establish the role of individual factors (e.g., lack of guilt feelings) for each group. For instance, are homicide offenders early in life already more aberrant than homicide victims in terms of callousness or lack of guilt feelings?

Childhood Predictors of Homicide Victims

Prevalence. In Chap. 3, we explained that there were 39 homicide victims in the Pittsburgh Youth Study. Not surprisingly in light of national statistics, African American males were more likely than Caucasian males to be homicide victims. Table 6.1 shows that 37 of the 39 victims (95%) were African American, compared with 765 of the 1,406 controls (54%). For comparability, the same 1,406 controls are used here as in Chap. 4. Prospectively, 4.3% of African American males were killed, compared with 0.3% of Caucasian males. Weighting back to the population of Pittsburgh public schools, 3.7% of African American males were killed, compared with 0.3% of Caucasian males. As mentioned, unweighted data are used in this book for the prediction analyses.

Table 6.1 Features of homicide victims

Feature	Percentage of controls (1,406)	Percentage of victims (39)	Odds ratio victims	Odds ratio offenders
African American	54	95	15.5*	5.4*
Weapon carrying	11	19	1.9	5.4*
Gun carrying	6	24	5.1*	3.4*
Used weapon	8	24	3.6*	3.9*
Gang member	14	21	1.7	2.5*
Gang fighting	5	20	4.6*	5.0*
Persistent drug user	19	21	1.2	2.6*
Sold marijuana	8	21	2.9*	3.6*
Sold hard drugs	8	24	3.9*	4.6*
Violence	46	82	5.3*	20.2*

Note: $*p < .05$

Antisocial Behavior. Table 6.1 also shows the extent to which homicide victims engaged in typical antisocial behaviors associated with delinquency (guns, gangs, and drugs), discussed in Chap. 5. These features were measured in multiple data waves (1–13 for the youngest cohort, up to age 15; 1–7 for the middle cohort, up to age 13; 1–7 for the oldest cohort, up to age 16) before any male became a homicide victim. Because of the focus on early childhood predictors, these antisocial behaviors are not studied as early risk factors in this chapter. Homicide victims compared to controls were significantly likely to have carried a gun, to have used a weapon (e.g., when attacking someone or in a gang fight or robbery), to have been involved in a gang fight, and to have sold marijuana or hard drugs. Thus, the majority of homicide victims were heavily engaged in a range of delinquent activities prior to being killed.

Table 6.1 shows that homicide victims were similar to convicted homicide offenders in carrying a gun, using a weapon, gang fighting, selling marijuana, and selling hard drugs. However, unlike convicted homicide offenders, homicide victims were not significantly likely to be gang members, persistent drug users, or to have carried a weapon. As mentioned, 32 of the 39 homicide victims (82%) were violent earlier in their life, compared with 652 of the 1,406 control boys (46%) (OR=5.3, CI=2.3–12.1; see Table 6.1). The comparable OR for convicted homicide offenders was 20.2 (CI=4.8–84.5).

Explanatory Predictors

In order to identify the predictors of homicide victims, we compared the 39 homicide victims with the 1,406 control boys. The same 21 explanatory and 19 behavioral risk factors used in Chap. 4 to predict homicide offenders were included in the analyses to predict homicide victims.

For ease of exposition, this chapter presents retrospective rather than prospective percentages. For example, Table 6.1 shows that 95% of homicide victims were

Table 6.2 Explanatory predictors of homicide victims

	Percentage of controls (1,406)	Percentage of victims (39)	Odds ratio	Partial OR	p
Lack of guilt	24	62	5.0*	4.5	.0001
Broken family	62	87	4.1*	3.1	.035
Low achievement (CAT)	24	51	3.4*	2.3	.016
HIA	17	36	2.7*	–	–
Old for the grade	25	46	2.6*	–	–
Low achievement (PT)	24	44	2.5*	–	–
Father behavior problems	17	33	2.5*	–	–
Large family size	21	38	2.3*	2.3	.023
Family on welfare	43	62	2.2*	–	–
Bad neighborhood (P)	24	41	2.2*	–	–
Bad neighborhood (C)	32	49	2.0*	–	–
Callous-unemotional	24	38	2.0	–	–

Notes: *CAT* California Achievement Test; *HIA* hyperactivity–impulsivity–attention deficit; *P* parent; *T* teacher; *C* census
*$p < .05$

African American, compared with 54% of controls. The OR for race vs. homicide victims was 15.5 (CI = 3.7–64.6). The confidence interval was large because of the small numbers of homicide victims.

Table 6.2 shows that 11 of the 21 explanatory factors significantly predicted homicide victims: lack of guilt, broken home, low achievement (according to the California Achievement Test), hyperactivity–impulsivity–attention deficit, old for the grade, low achievement (according to mother–teacher ratings), behavior problems of the father, large family size, the family on welfare, and bad neighborhood according to census data and mother ratings. In addition, callous-unemotional behavior was almost significant as a predictor. The strongest predictor was lack of guilt: 62% of homicide victims lacked guilt, compared with 24% of controls (OR = 5.0, CI = 2.6–9.6).

Explanatory Risk Score. A logistic regression analysis was carried out to investigate which of the 11 significant explanatory predictors of homicide victims were independent predictors. Four variables were significant in a stepwise regression analysis: lack of guilt (LRCS = 26.88, $p < .0001$), low achievement on the CAT (LRCS = 6.64, $p = .010$), a broken home (LRCS = 5.74, $p = .017$), and large family size (LRCS = 5.57, $p = .018$). In the final model, the partial odds ratios were 4.5 for lack of guilt, 3.1 for broken family, 2.3 for low achievement, and 2.3 for large family size. These partial odds ratios are shown in Table 6.2. The results suggest that individual, family, and school factors all contributed to the explanation and prediction of homicide victims.

Next we calculated an explanatory risk score for each boy based on the number of these four risk factors that he was exposed to in childhood. Figure 6.1 shows a steadily increasing dose–response relationship between the explanatory risk score and the probability of becoming a homicide victim. Only 0.6% of 333 boys with none of these four risk factors became homicide victims, compared with 8.9% of 235

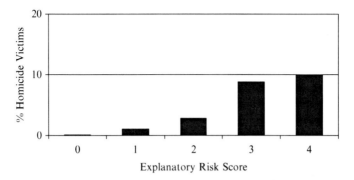

Fig. 6.1 Explanatory risk score predicting homicide victims

boys with three or four of these risk factors. Retrospectively, 21 of the 39 homicide victims (54%) were among the one-sixth of the boys with three or four of these risk factors. Comparing boys with 0–2 risk factors with those with 3–4 risk factors produced an OR = 6.5 (CI = 3.4–12.3). The AUC = .768 (SD = .037). This was higher than the AUC for the prediction of convicted homicide offenders on the basis of an explanatory risk score (AUC = .735; Fig. 4.1). Therefore, the prediction of homicide victims on the basis of explanatory factors was, if anything, slightly more accurate than the prediction of homicide offenders.

Comparing Victims and Offenders. Did homicide victims compared to homicide offenders grow up under less deprived conditions or exposed to fewer risk factors? Based on explanatory risk factors, homicide offenders were not more extreme than homicide victims; the 11 significant predictors for victims could be compared with 9 significant predictors for offenders. Five factors significantly predicted both offenders and victims: old for the grade, lack of guilt, the family on welfare, a broken home, and a bad neighborhood according to census data. However, it was noteworthy that the strongest predictors of homicide offenders were mostly socioeconomic/demographic factors: five of the strongest six predictors were a broken home, a bad neighborhood according to census data, the family on welfare, a young mother, and an unemployed mother. In contrast, the strongest predictors of homicide victims were mostly individual factors: five of the strongest seven predictors were lack of guilt and several school factors, including low achievement (according to both the CAT and mother–teacher ratings), hyperactivity–impulsivity–attention deficit, and old for the grade (held back in school).

Why does Race Predict Homicide Victims? In Table 6.1, we showed that the majority of the homicide victims were African American. It is plausible to suggest that race predicts homicide victims because African American and Caucasian boys differ on predictive risk factors. According to this hypothesis, race should not predict homicide victims after controlling for such risk factors. However, after entering the 11 significant explanatory risk factors in a logistic regression analysis, race was still a significant predictor of homicide victims (LRCS = 14.88, p = .0001). Further exploration of the data suggested that the predictability of race for homicide victims held up after controlling for all other explanatory variables. This is not surprising, in light of the fact that 37 of the 39 homicide victims were African American.

Nevertheless, we still believe that race predicts homicide victims because African American boys were more deprived than Caucasian boys on socioeconomic/demographic factors such as broken home, the family on welfare, a bad neighborhood, and a young mother, as indeed we found in Chap. 4 for the prediction of convicted homicide offenders. Other analyses of Pittsburgh data (Farrington, Loeber, & Stouthamer-Loeber, 2003; Huizinga et al., 2006) have also shown that, once other social and structural factors are taken into account, race does not predict violence. Later in this chapter, we review the extent to which race predicts shooting victims.

Behavioral Predictors

Fourteen of the 19 behavioral factors significantly predicted homicide victims: serious delinquency, physical and nonphysical aggression, a bad relationship with a parent, covert behavior, a high-risk score, a bad relationship with peers, suspended from school, bad friends, low school motivation, cruel to people, peer delinquency, truancy, and disruptive behavior disorder (Table 6.3). The strongest predictor was serious delinquency: 67% of homicide victims had been serious delinquents, compared with 29% of controls (OR = 5.0, CI = 2.5–9.8).

Table 6.3 Behavioral predictors of homicide victims

	Percentage of controls (1,406)	Percentage of victims (39)	Odds ratio	Partial OR	p
Serious delinquency	29	67	5.0*	3.5	.0006
Physical aggression	26	56	3.6*	2.0	.050
Nonphysical aggression	25	54	3.5*	–	–
Bad relationship with parent	24	51	3.3*	2.2	.024
Covert behavior	24	50	3.1*	–	–
High-risk score	49	74	3.0*	–	–
Bad relationship with peers	26	49	2.7*	–	–
Suspended	43	66	2.6*	–	–
Bad friends	25	46	2.6*	–	–
Low school motivation	37	59	2.5*	–	–
Cruel to people	24	44	2.4*	–	–
Peer delinquency	24	41	2.2*	–	–
Truant	38	56	2.1*	–	–
Disruptive behavior disorder	23	37	2.0*	–	–

Note: *$p < .05$

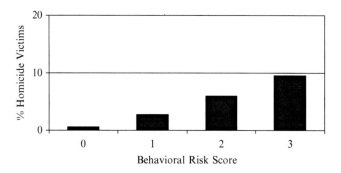

Fig. 6.2 Behavioral risk score predicting homicide victims

Behavioral Risk Score. A logistic regression analysis was carried out to investigate which of the 14 significant predictors of homicide victims were independent predictors. Three variables were significant in a stepwise analysis: serious delinquency (LRCS = 23.26, $p < .0001$), a bad relationship with a parent (LRCS = 7.35, $p = .007$), and physical aggression (LRCS = 3.89, $p = .048$). In the final model, the partial odds ratios were 3.5 for serious delinquency, 2.2 for a bad relationship with a parent, and 2.0 for physical aggression (Table 6.3). Thus, the combination of serious property offenses, physical aggression and a poor relationship with parents was the most important childhood precursor of homicide victims.

A behavioral risk score was then calculated for each boy based on the number of these three risk factors that he possessed. Figure 6.2 shows a dose–response relationship: the higher the behavioral risk score, the higher the probability of becoming a homicide victim. For example, 0.6% of 702 boys with none of these three risk factors became homicide victims, compared with 9.5% of 95 boys with all three of these risk factors. Retrospectively, 24 of the 39 homicide victims (62%) were among the quarter of the boys with two or three of these risk factors. Comparing boys with 0–1 risk factors with those with 2–3 risk factors, OR = 5.5 (CI = 2.8–10.5); comparing boys with 0–2 risk factors with those with all 3 risk factors, OR = 4.6 (CI = 2.1–10.0). The AUC was .780 (SD = .034). The behavioral prediction of homicide victims was at least as accurate as the behavioral prediction of homicide offenders (AUC = 773; Fig. 4.2).

Comparing Victims and Offenders. There were 11 significant behavioral predictors of convicted homicide offenders and 14 significant behavioral predictors of homicide victims. Nine factors significantly predicted both: a high-risk score, truancy, serious delinquency, covert behavior, suspended from school, cruel to people, peer delinquency, bad friends, and disruptive behavior disorder. Homicide offenders were not more extreme than homicide victims; in fact, there were more significant results in predicting victims than in predicting offenders. These results suggest that young homicide offenders were not more antisocial than young homicide victims.

Screening Risk Score. As pointed out in previous chapters, predictive efficiency is overestimated in the above analyses because the risk score is calculated in light of

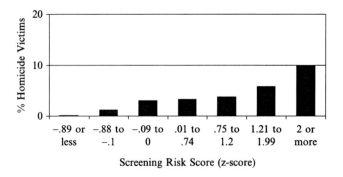

Fig. 6.3 Screening risk score predicting homicide victims

knowledge about which risk factors were the best predictors of homicide victims. In order to derive a more accurate estimate of predictive efficiency, the screening risk score was used.

Figure 6.3 shows the dose–response relationship between the screening risk score and the percentage of homicide victims, which increased from 0.8% of those with the lowest Z-scores to 9.8% of those with the highest Z-scores. Retrospectively, 17 of the 38 homicide victims (45%; one was not known on the screening risk score) were among the one-fifth of boys in the top three categories (Z-score .75 or greater). Comparing boys in these categories with the remainder, OR = 3.1 (CI=1.6–5.9). The AUC was .707 (SD = .042), almost identical to the comparable AUC for predicting convicted homicide offenders.

Comparing results from the screening risk score with those from the behavioral risk score, the AUC decreased from .780 to .707, as in the results for predicting convicted homicide offenders. The most comparable OR decreased from 5.5 to 3.1 (CI=1.6–5.9). As explained before, part of this decrease is attributable to the more limited predictor (only one variable) and part probably reflects the overestimation of predictive efficiency by the behavioral risk score. It is reasonable to suggest that an unbiased AUC based on a behavioral risk score might be of the order of .72–.75, that an unbiased OR might be of the order of 4, and that about 6–7% of the worst one-fifth of the sample might become homicide victims, including over 40% of all homicide victims.

Criminal Predictors

Previous research suggests that homicide victims often have extensive criminal histories (e.g., Brodie, Daday, Crandall, Sklar, & Jost, 2006; Dobrin, 2001). To what extent can homicide victims be predicted on the basis of their prior criminal histories? In order to investigate this question, convictions, arrests, and self-reports of offending up to age 14 were studied (described in Chap. 4). All prior crimes occurred before any boy was killed. As before, 39 homicide victims were compared with 1,406 control boys.

Table 6.4 Criminal predictors of homicide victims

	Percentage of controls (1,406)	Percentage of victims (39)	Odds ratio
Self-reports			
Vehicle theft	12	38	4.5*
Aggravated assault	13	36	3.9*
Theft from car	13	36	3.8*
Receiving	15	41	3.8*
Violence (3)	28	56	3.3*
Theft (4)	27	51	2.9*
Drug selling	8	18	2.7*
Arson	12	26	2.5*
Gang fight	23	41	2.4*
Drunk in public	9	18	2.3*
Marijuana use	15	28	2.2*
Minor fraud	46	64	2.1*
Vandalism	53	69	2.0*
Convictions			
Drug	1	8	7.7*
Vehicle theft	5	21	4.9*
Receiving	6	23	4.8*
Theft (3)	10	31	4.2*
Other/conspiracy	11	33	4.0*
Any conviction	17	44	3.8*
Larceny	5	13	3.1*
Arrests			
Receiving	10	41	6.1*
Vehicle theft	7	31	5.7*
Drug	2	10	5.4*
Other/conspiracy	17	51	5.0*
Theft (3)	15	44	4.4*
Mischief/disorder	6	21	4.2*
Robbery	3	10	3.6*
Any arrest	28	56	3.4*
Larceny	10	26	3.2*
Simple assault	7	18	3.0*
Violence (3)	11	26	2.7*

Note: *$p < .05$
For definition of variables see Tables 4.4, 4.5, 4.6

Table 6.4 summarizes the strongest criminal predictors of homicide victims. For self-reports, the strongest predictor was vehicle theft: 38% of victims had stolen a vehicle up to age 14, compared with 12% of controls (OR=4.5, CI=2.3–8.7). Interestingly, self-reported vehicle theft was also the strongest predictor of convicted homicide offenders (Table 4.4). Aggravated assault, theft from a car, and receiving stolen property were also strong predictors of homicide victims.

For convictions, the strongest predictors of homicide victims were drug offenses, vehicle theft, and receiving stolen property. In total, 17 of the 39 victims (44%) were convicted up to age 14, compared with 17% of the 1,406 controls (OR=3.8,

Table 6.5 Logistic regression analyses for criminal predictors

Based on:	LRCS	p	Partial OR	p
Self-reports				
Vehicle theft	16.79	.0001	2.4	.028
Aggravated assault	5.21	.022	2.1	.042
Receiving	3.75	.053	2.1	.048
Convictions				
Receiving	12.07	.0005	2.3	.093
Drug	3.55	.060	3.7	.051
Other/conspiracy	3.53	.060	2.4	.049
Arrests				
Receiving	24.20	.0001	3.1	.012
Other/conspiracy	4.55	.033	2.6	.028
All				
Receiving (A)	23.67	.0001	3.9	.0002
Aggravated assault (S)	8.10	.004	2.4	.019
Receiving (S)	3.75	.053	2.1	.042
Drug (C)	3.05	.081	3.9	.050

Notes: *(A)* arrests, *(S)* self-reports, *(C)* convictions, *LRCS* likelihood ratio chi-squared, *OR* odds ratio

$CI = 2.0–7.2$). For arrests, the strongest predictors of homicide victims were receiving stolen property, vehicle theft, and drug offenses. In total, 22 of the 39 victims (56%) were arrested up to age 14, compared with 28% of the 1,406 controls ($OR = 3.4$, $CI = 1.8–6.4$). Prior convictions and arrests predicted convicted homicide offenders more strongly than homicide victims (compare Tables 4.5 and 4.6). Summarizing the analyses for the three types of delinquency information, the results show the predominance of property offenses that predicted homicide victims, including receiving stolen goods (three significant results) and vehicle theft (three significant results).

Criminal Risk Score. Logistic regression analyses were carried out to investigate which types of prior offenses up to age 14 independently predicted later homicide victims. Separate analyses were carried out for self-reports, convictions, and arrests. All significant offense variables were entered into the regressions. Table 6.5 shows the results. Self-reported vehicle theft, aggravated assault, and receiving stolen property independently predicted later homicide victims. Convictions for receiving stolen property, drug offenses, and other/conspiracy were also independent predictors, as were arrests for receiving and other/conspiracy.

All of these eight variables were then entered into a final logistic regression analysis to establish the independent predictors from all of the self-report, conviction, and arrest information up to age 14. Table 6.5 shows the results. Four variables were significant independent predictors: arrests for receiving, self-reports of aggravated assaults and receiving, and convictions for drug offenses.

A criminal risk score was then calculated based on the number of these four criminal risk factors that each boy possessed. Figure 6.4 shows a dose–response relationship between the criminal risk score and the probability of becoming a homicide victim.

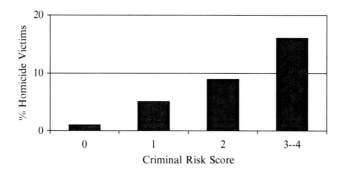

Fig. 6.4 Criminal risk score predicting homicide victims

Only 1% of boys with none of these risk factors became homicide victims, compared with 9% of those with two risk factors and 16% of those with three or four risk factors. A total of 143 boys (10%) possessed two, three, or four risk factors, and 15 of them became homicide victims (10%), compared with 2% of the remaining 1,302 boys. This cutoff point identified 38% of the homicide victims. The AUC of .806 (SD = .036) for criminal risk factors was somewhat higher than for explanatory (AUC = .768) or behavioral (AUC = .780) risk factors, but lower than for the prediction of convicted homicide offenders by criminal risk factors (AUC = .837; Fig. 4.4). The OR for a cutoff point of two or more risk factors was 6.2 (CI = 3.2–12.2), compared with an OR of 7.8 (CI = 2.8–21.6) for a cutoff of three or more risk factors.

Comparing Victims and Offenders. The strongest self-report predictor of homicide victims was vehicle theft, which was also the strongest self-report predictor of convicted homicide offenders. Similarly, other/conspiracy convictions and other/conspiracy arrests were among the strongest predictors of both victims and offenders. Other criminal predictors were different. Nevertheless, it is clear that homicide victims, like convicted homicide offenders, had extensive prior criminal records.

The Use of Arrest in Estimating True Prediction. As before, it might be argued that predictive accuracy is overestimated in the analysis of criminal risk scores, because the constituent variables are chosen in light of knowledge about which are the best predictors. In order to produce a more realistic estimate of predictive efficiency, the number of arrests up to age 14 was used.

Figure 6.5 shows the extent to which the number of arrests up to age 14 predicted homicide victims. Of 94 boys with nine or more arrests, ten (11%) became victims, compared with 2% of the 1,351 boys with fewer arrests (OR = 5.4; CI = 2.6–11.5). However, only 10 of the 39 victims (26%) were identified by this cutoff point. Of 187 boys with five or more arrests, 17 (9%) became victims, compared with 2% of the 1,258 boys with fewer arrests (OR = 5.6; CI = 2.9–10.8). This cutoff point identified 44% of the 39 victims. The odds ratios and AUC were lower here than for the prediction of convicted homicide offenders.

The AUC for the number of arrests was .706 (SD = .062), compared with .806 for the criminal risk score. It is reasonable to suggest that an unbiased AUC based on a

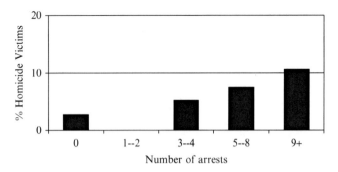

Fig. 6.5 Number of arrests up to age 14 predicting homicide victims

criminal risk score might be of the order of .75, that an unbiased OR might be about 6, and that about 9–10% of the worst one-eighth of the sample might become homicide victims, including over 40% of all homicide victims.

Integrated Prediction of Homicide Victims

In the final exercise to predict homicide victims, all the significant, independently predictive risk factors (explanatory, behavioral, and criminal) from Tables 6.2–6.5 were entered into a logistic regression analysis. Table 6.6 shows the results. The following six risk factors independently predicted homicide victims: lack of guilt, an arrest for receiving stolen property, aggravated assault according to self-reports, low achievement (according to the California Achievement Test), large family size, and a bad relationship with a parent. All of these factors were recorded up to age 14, and it is interesting that four of the best six predictors were explanatory variables. In summary, early offending in combination with poor school factors and disadvantaged family factors all contributed to the prediction of homicide victims.

Integrated Homicide Victim Risk Score. Is there a dose–response relationship between the number of risk factors and the probability of becoming a homicide victim? To address this question, we computed an integrated homicide victim risk score using information from the final regression analysis, which allowed us to compute a final risk score based on the number of the six risk factors that each boy possessed. Figure 6.6 shows a positively accelerating dose–response relationship between the integrated risk score and the probability of becoming a homicide victim. Only 4 out of 950 boys scoring 0 or 1 (0.4%) became homicide victims, compared with 12 out of 70 scoring 4–6 (17%) (OR = 10.3, CI=5.0–21.4). A total of 220 boys (15%) possessed three or more of these risk factors, and 23 of them (10%) became homicide victims, compared with 1% of the remaining 1,222 boys (OR=8.8, CI=4.6–17.0). This cutoff point identified 59% of the homicide victims. The final AUC of .840 (SD=.027) was higher than for any of the constituent scales but some

Table 6.6 Final logistic regression analysis predicting homicide victims

Predictors	LRCS	p	Partial OR	p
Lack of guilt	26.55	.0001	3.9	.0002
Receiving (arrest)	11.87	.0006	3.2	.003
Aggravated assault (self-report)	6.89	.009	2.5	.018
Low achievement (CAT)	4.56	.033	2.2	.032
Large family size	4.46	.035	2.2	.027
Bad relationship with parent	4.44	.035	2.2	.033

Notes: LRCS likelihood ratio chi-squared, *OR* odds ratio, *CAT* California Achievement Test

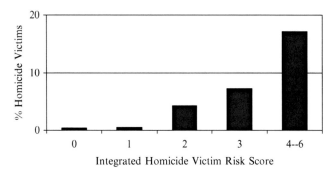

Fig. 6.6 Integrated homicide victim risk score predicting homicide victims

what lower than for the prediction of convicted homicide offenders (AUC=.870, Chap. 4). Nevertheless, it is clear from all the analyses in this chapter that the explanatory, behavioral, and criminal risk factors generally predict homicide victims about as well as homicide offenders.

Shooting Victims

Homicide victims are a tragic subgroup of a larger population who are victims of shootings. Of the 1,517 boys in the sample, 128 (8.4%) were shot before age 30. Weighting back to the population, 7.6% of Pittsburgh public school boys were shot before age 30, including 1.3% of Caucasian boys and 12.6% of African American boys. As with the homicide victims, information about shooting victims came from the boys and their families, and from newspaper reports. Of the 128 shooting victims, 37 died, 9 were arrested for homicide, and 6 were convicted for homicide.

Of the 1,406 control boys in this chapter, 78 (5.5%) were shooting victims (who did not die and were not arrested or convicted), and these are compared with the remaining 1,328 control boys. Of the 78 shooting victims, 90% were African American, compared with 52% of the control boys in this analysis (OR=8.0, CI=3.8–16.7).

Table 6.7 Features of shooting victims

Feature	Percentage of controls (1,328)	Percentage of victims (78)	Odds ratio
African American	52	90	8.0*
Weapon carrying	11	9	0.7
Gun carrying	6	14	2.9*
Used weapon	8	13	1.8
Gang member	13	40	4.5*
Gang fighting	5	4	0.8
Persistent drug user	18	27	1.7
Sold marijuana	8	20	2.9*
Sold hard drugs	6	28	5.7*

Note: $*p < .05$

Table 6.7 shows that the shooting victims were significantly more likely than the controls to have been antisocial. More of the shooting victims compared to controls had sold hard drugs (OR=5.7, CI=3.2–10.0), were gang members (OR=4.5, CI=2.7–7.6), carried a gun (OR=2.9, CI=1.4–5.8), and had sold marijuana (OR=2.9, CI=1.6–5.4). Next, we addressed the following question: *Are homicide victims and shooting victims similar in their antisocial behavior?* A comparison of Tables 6.1 and 6.7 shows that the homicide victims were similar to the shooting victims in antisocial behaviors, including selling hard drugs and marijuana and in carrying a gun. However, unlike the shooting victims, the homicide victims did not tend to be gang members.

Explanatory Predictors. Fifteen of the 21 explanatory factors significantly predicted shooting victims compared with controls (see Table 6.8). The strongest predictors were a broken home, a bad neighborhood according to census data, callous-unemotional behavior, the family on welfare, behavior problems of the father, and an unemployed mother. The independently important factors were a broken home, an unemployed mother, and hyperactivity–impulsivity–attention deficit. Overall, the results show that predictors of shooting victims overlapped with predictors of homicide victims. Ten of the 12 strongest explanatory predictors of homicide victims (Table 6.2) were among the 15 strongest predictors of shooting victims.

Why Does Race Predict Shooting Victims? As mentioned, 90% of the shooting victims (70 out of 78) were African American. It is plausible to suggest that race predicts shooting victims because African American and Caucasian boys differ on predictive risk factors. According to this hypothesis, race should not predict shooting victims after controlling for such risk factors. However, after entering the 15 significant explanatory risk factors in a logistic regression analysis, race was still a significant predictor of shooting victims (LRCS=6.62, p=.010). Nevertheless, the predictive power of race was greatly reduced after controlling for explanatory risk factors, from the original OR of 8.0 to a partial OR of 3.5. Therefore, it is reasonable to conclude that much of the relationship between race and shooting victims is explained by differences in risk factors between African American and Caucasian boys.

Table 6.8 Explanatory predictors of shooting victims

	Percentage of controls (1,328)	Percentage of victims (78)	Odds ratio	Partial OR	p
Broken family	61	87	4.3*	3.7	.0002
Bad neighborhood (C)	31	56	2.9*	–	–
Callous-unemotional	23	41	2.3*	–	–
Family on welfare	42	63	2.3*	–	–
Father behavior problems	16	30	2.2*	–	–
Unemployed mother	24	40	2.2*	1.8	.020
Low achievement (CAT)	23	39	2.1*	–	–
HIA	17	28	2.0*	1.9	.017
Depressed mood	22	36	2.0*	–	–
Low socioeconomic status	25	40	2.0*	–	–
Low achievement (PT)	23	37	2.0*	–	–
Young mother	20	32	1.9*	–	–
Lack of guilt	24	36	1.8*	–	–
Parent substance use	27	38	1.7*	–	–
Bad neighborhood (P)	24	34	1.6*	–	–

Notes: *$p<.05$
OR odds ratio, *P* parent, *T* teacher, *C* census, *HIA* hyperactivity–impulsivity–attention deficit, CAT California Achievement Test

Table 6.9 Behavioral predictors of shooting victims

	Percentage of controls (1,328)	Percentage of victims (78)	Odds ratio	Partial OR	p
Suspended	42	63	2.4*	–	–
Truant	36	58	2.4*	1.9	.017
Peer delinquency	23	41	2.4*	1.9	.019
Low school motivation	35	57	2.4*	2.4	.002
Serious delinquency	28	46	2.2*	–	–
Bad relationship with peers	25	41	2.1*	–	–
High-risk score	48	65	2.0*	–	–
Cruel to people	24	38	2.0*	–	–
Covert behavior	23	37	1.9*	–	–
Physical aggression	26	36	1.6*	–	–

Notes: *$p<.05$; *OR* odds ratio

Behavioral Predictors. Ten of the 19 behavioral (and attitudinal) factors significantly predicted shooting victims (see Table 6.9). The strongest predictors were suspended from school, truant, peer delinquency, low school motivation, and serious delinquency. The independent predictors were truant, peer delinquency, and low school motivation. The predictors of shooting victims overlapped considerably with the predictors of homicide victims. All 10 of the behavioral factors in Table 6.9 were among the 13 strongest behavioral predictors of homicide victims in Table 6.3.

Table 6.10 Criminal predictors of shooting victims

	Percentage of controls (1,328)	Percentage of victims (78)	Odds ratio	Partial OR	p
Mischief/disorder (C)	2	9	4.0*	2.6	.045
Drug selling (S)	7	21	3.8*	1.9	.062
Gang fight (S)	21	49	3.7*	2.5	.0007
Aggravated assault (C)	2	8	3.6*	–	–
Vehicle theft (S)	11	25	2.6*	–	–
Aggravated assault (A)	4	9	2.5*	–	–
Receiving (S)	15	29	2.4*	–	–
Marijuana use (S)	15	29	2.4*	–	–
Minor fraud (S)	45	67	2.4*	1.7	.060
Drunk in public (S)	8	17	2.4*	–	–
Vehicle theft (A)	7	14	2.3*	–	–
Mischief/disorder (A)	5	12	2.3*	–	–
Burglary (S)	13	24	2.2*	–	–
Weapon carrying (S)	39	55	2.0*	–	–
Shoplifting (S)	45	60	1.8*	–	–
Other theft (S)	43	57	1.7*	–	–

Notes: *$p < .05$; (C) conviction, (A) arrest, (S) self-report

Criminal Predictors. Table 6.10 shows the 16 significant criminal predictors of shooting victims, based on convictions, arrests, and self-reports of offending up to age 14. The strongest predictors were convictions for mischief/disorder and aggravated assault, and self-reports of drug selling and gang fighting. The independent predictors were convictions for mischief/disorder, and self-report of drug selling, gang fighting, and minor fraud. Once again, the predictors of shooting victims overlapped considerably with the predictors of homicide victims. Nine of the 16 significant criminal predictors of shooting victims (Table 6.10) were also significant predictors of homicide victims (Table 6.5): arrests for vehicle theft and mischief/disorder, and self-reports of drug selling, gang fighting, vehicle theft, receiving stolen property, marijuana use, minor fraud, and drunk in public.

Integrated Shooting Victim Risk Score. The ten independent predictors identified in Tables 6.8–6.10 were included in a final logistic regression analysis to establish the strongest independent predictors, from all three domains, of shooting victims. The five most important predictors were: a broken home (partial OR = 3.4, $p < .0001$), self-reported drug selling (partial OR = 3.0, $p = .001$), low school motivation (partial OR = 1.8, $p = .035$), truant (partial OR = 1.7, $p = .052$), and peer delinquency (partial OR = 1.6, $p = .085$).

An integrated shooting victim risk score was calculated based on the number of these five risk factors that each boy possessed. Figure 6.7 shows a dose–response relationship: the higher the integrated risk score, the higher the probability of becoming a shooting victim. Less than 1% of boys with none of these risk factors became shooting victims, compared with 10% of boys with three risk factors and 15% of boys with four or five risk factors. A total of 423 boys (30%) possessed

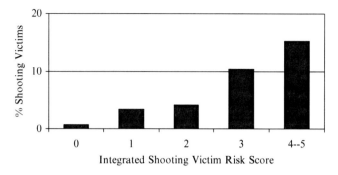

Fig. 6.7 Integrated shooting victim risk score predicting shooting victims

3–5 risk factors, and 50 of them (12%) became shooting victims, compared with 2% of the remaining 979 boys (OR = 4.6, CI=2.8–7.3). This cutoff point identified 64% of the shooting victims.

Comparison Between Homicide Victims and Shooting Victims. On the one hand, there is a large chance element in who is killed compared to those wounded as a result of a confrontation, and homicide victims and shooting victims may actually have similar deviant backgrounds. On the other hand, it might be expected that homicide victims are more extreme in their behavior than shooting victims. Therefore, we addressed the following question: *Do early risk factors predict homicide victims more accurately than shooting victims?* The AUC of .733 (SD = .028) for predicting shooting victims was lower than the corresponding AUC of .840 for predicting homicide victims, and the ORs were also lower for shooting victims (OR = 3.7 for a cutoff of four or more risk factors; OR = 4.6 for a cutoff of three or more risk factors). This suggests that shooting victims were predicted less accurately than were homicide victims.

Conclusions

This is the first prospective longitudinal study of characteristics of homicide and shooting victims. However, it has a number of limitations. In particular, the numbers of homicide and shooting victims were small, and results obtained in the City of Pittsburgh may not be generalizable to the USA.

Nevertheless, this chapter shows that childhood explanatory and behavioral risk factors measured in the PYS significantly predicted homicide victims up to 22 years later. Behavioral risk factors were only slightly better predictors than explanatory risk factors. Importantly, homicide victims were at least as deviant as homicide offenders, and victims were generally predicted as accurately as offenders. For example, 57% of homicide offenders and 67% of homicide victims had already committed serious delinquency (burglary, vehicle theft, robbery, assault, or rape), compared with 29% of controls. Like homicide offenders, homicide victims tended to have carried and used a weapon, to have sold drugs, and to have been involved in gang fighting.

The strongest predictors of homicide offenders tended also to be the strongest predictors of homicide victims. However, among the significant explanatory predictors, homicide offenders tended to be predicted more by sociodemographic factors (e.g., a broken home, a young or unemployed mother, a bad neighborhood, the family on welfare) and homicide victims tended to be predicted more by individual factors (e.g., lack of guilt, low achievement, hyperactivity). Thus, victims tended to be more individually deviant while offenders tended to be more socially deprived. Coming from a broken home was one of the most important predictors of both homicide offenders and victims. African American boys were more likely to be both offenders and victims, but much of this race difference was explainable by race differences in risk factors.

Risk scores showed how much homicide victims could be predicted in the first year of the PYS. Typically, less than 1% of the least risky boys, compared to 7–10% of the most risky boys, became homicide victims. In an unbiased prediction based on the screening risk score, about 6–7% of the worst one-fifth of the sample became homicide victims, including over 40% of all homicide victims.

One possible interpretation of these results is that multiple early risk factors (including socioeconomic deprivation and low school attainment) cause an antisocial lifestyle involving guns, gangs, and drugs, that increases the risk of being involved in a homicide either as an offender or as a victim. Further research is needed to test this theory and to investigate why sociodemographic factors are more important for homicide offenders while individual factors are more important for homicide victims.

Early offending also predicted homicide victims; 56% of them had been arrested and 44% had been convicted up to age 14. The types of offenses that were most characteristic of homicide victims were vehicle theft, aggravated assault, receiving stolen property, drug offenses, and other/conspiracy. It was interesting that vehicle theft and receiving stolen property were so important in the early criminal histories of homicide victims. Criminal risk scores showed that only 1% of the least risky boys, compared with 16% of the most risky boys, became homicide victims. In an unbiased analysis based on the number of arrests, about 9–10% of the worst one-eighth of the sample became homicide victims, including over 40% of all homicide victims.

In an analysis of explanatory, behavioral, and criminal risk factors, the independent predictors of homicide victims included four explanatory variables (lack of guilt, low achievement, large family size, and a bad relationship with a parent) and two criminal variables (an arrest for receiving stolen property and a self-report of aggravated assault). It was interesting that early explanatory variables were still important after controlling for behavioral and criminal factors. Only 0.5% of the least risky boys, according to these six variables, became homicide victims, compared with 17% of the most risky boys.

Turning to shooting victims, the most important explanatory predictors were a broken home, a bad neighborhood, callous-unemotional behavior, and the family on welfare. The strongest behavioral predictors were suspended from school, truant, peer delinquency, and low school motivation. The strongest criminal predictors were convictions for mischief/disorder and aggravated assault, and self-reports of drug selling and gang fighting. In general, the strongest predictors of shooting victims were similar to the strongest predictors of homicide victims. Like homicide victims, shooting victims tended to have carried a gun, to be involved in gangs, and to have sold drugs.

In an analysis of explanatory, behavioral, and criminal risk factors, the independent predictors of shooting victims were a broken home, self-reported drug selling, low school motivation, truant, and peer delinquency. Less than 1% of the least risky boys, according to these five variables, became shooting victims, compared with 12% of the most risky boys. However, shooting victims were predicted less well by these risk factors than were homicide offenders.

It is clear that early risk factors can be used to identify boys with very different probabilities of becoming homicide victims and shooting victims. Interestingly, in most analyses, homicide victims were predicted just as efficiently as homicide offenders. These results could be used to develop and test risk assessment instruments.

Chapter 7
Homicide Offenders Speak

Darrick Jolliffe, Rolf Loeber, David P. Farrington, and Robert B. Cotter

Chapter 4 summarized childhood predictors of homicide offenders, while Chap. 5 reviewed predictors of homicide offenders among violent offenders. Most of the predictors that were included in these prediction exercises were evident many years prior to the homicide offense. We now turn to more proximal circumstances that probably influenced why some individuals and not others committed homicide. Some of these are reviewed in Chap. 3. To study these proximal factors in more detail, we undertook face-to-face interviews with the convicted homicide offenders, together with matched controls.

The purpose of this chapter is to test several hypotheses. As in the work of Loeber et al. (2005a), we hypothesize that those convicted of homicide will present as more extreme in terms of risk factors compared to matched controls. We are particularly keen to establish whether homicide offenders compared to controls score higher on indicators of serious delinquency, gang membership, heavy substance use, and psychopathy.

A second hypothesis is that proximal circumstances will distinguish the homicide offenders and their controls. To address this hypothesis, we will examine situational aspects of homicide such as the reason for the offense, its setting and timing, weapon use, the assistance of co-offenders, drug and alcohol use prior to the offense, and the homicide offenders' knowledge of and feelings about the victim.

Methods

Attempts were made to interview the 33 homicide offenders who were convicted up to February 2006, and 27 were interviewed (82%). Three homicide offenders were incarcerated outside Pennsylvania. Attempts were made to contact each of these on four occasions by letter in order to obtain their consent to participate, but there was no response each time. One participant incarcerated in the Pennsylvania prison system also did not respond to repeated letters. Two participants had completed their prison sentences, but after exhaustive searches they could not be located.

R. Loeber and D.P. Farrington, *Young Homicide Offenders and Victims*,
Longitudinal Research in the Social and Behavioral Sciences: An Interdisciplinary Series,
DOI 10.1007/978-1-4419-9949-8_7, © Springer Science+Business Media, LLC 2011

For every convicted homicide offender who was interviewed, a matched control participant was also interviewed. Controls were sought for interviews only after the offender's interview was completed. Each control participant was matched with an offender based on the following criteria: (1) Race; (2) Birthday (±1 year); (3) Participant who lived in the same Census Tract as the offender at screening, and if this was not possible, participant who lived in the same Census Neighborhood as the offender at screening, or participant at screening who lived in a Census Tract with the same neighborhood disadvantage score based on information from the census (Wikström & Loeber, 2000). Of the possible matches, the participant with the closest birthday to the offender was selected. Due to refusals and participants not being located, the "best" match could not always be interviewed as a control: 13 controls were the best match, 6 were the second best match, 2 were the third best match, and 6 were the fourth best match. Therefore, there were 27 convicted homicide offenders and their 27 control participants.

Measures

The interviews focused on a number of key background characteristics which included basic demographic information, information about gang membership, information about drug use and self-reported delinquency, and an assessment of psychopathy (the time window for nonincarcerated individuals was the past year; the time window for incarcerated individuals was the year prior to the arrest leading to incarceration). Also, all homicide offenders described the situations that resulted in their offense, and as much as possible this was analyzed.

Incarceration. We distinguished between two groups of individuals based on whether or not they were incarcerated at the time of the study. As would be expected, a large proportion of those convicted of homicide (93%) were incarcerated at the time of the study. In contrast, only one of the homicide controls was incarcerated. Overall, those convicted of homicide were significantly more likely to be incarcerated than their controls (OR = 332.1, $p < .0001$).

This differential level of incarceration complicates comparisons of the convicted men and the controls. In an attempt to allow for this potential problem, questions were posed about "the past year, or the year prior to the arrest for your current offense." In this way, the influence of incarceration on the results was minimized. The disadvantage, however, is that recall may have been better for recent than for more distal events.

Results

Demographics. Table 7.1 shows some key demographic factors. The convicted men and controls were very similar in age (26–27). Those convicted of homicide were significantly less likely to be married at the time of the interview than controls

Table 7.1 Demographics of convicted homicide offenders and controls

	Convicted homicide offenders	Controls	Convicted vs. controls (OR)
Mean age	26.4	27.0	0.9
% Married	0	24	0.1*
% Ever lived as married	48	55	0.8
Mean no. of children	0.5	1.1	0.3*

Note: *p<.05

Table 7.2 Prevalence of self-reported offending of convicted homicide offenders and controls

Prevalence	Convicted homicide offenders (%)	Controls (%)	Convicted vs. controls (OR)
Moderate theft	51.9	3.7	26.2*
Serious theft	14.8	0	4.7*
Serious violence	74.1	7.4	37.6*
Drug dealing	88.9	3.7	192.5*

Note: *p<.05

(OR=0.1, $p<.0001$). None of the offenders was married. It is not clear whether this is a result of extended incarceration or whether the eventual homicide offenders had fewer permanent partners prior to committing homicide. In agreement with a lower proportion married, those convicted of homicide also reported having fewer children. These results may reflect the impact of incarceration rather than any real differences between those convicted of homicide and the controls. This is because, when asked if they had ever lived with someone as married, those convicted of homicide did not differ significantly from their controls.

Self-Reported Delinquency. Were the homicide offenders more extreme in their offending during the year prior to committing homicide? Table 7.2 shows the prevalence of self-reported offending. Moderate theft involved theft of $5 or greater, snatching a purse or wallet, and buying, holding, or selling stolen goods. Serious theft included breaking and entering and car theft. Serious violence included attack with a weapon, hitting with the intent of hurting, using weapons, force or strong-arm methods to obtain money or things, physically hurting or threatening to obtain sex, and having sex with someone against their will. The results showed that those convicted of homicide were significantly more likely than their controls to report moderate theft (OR=26.2, $p<.0001$), serious theft (OR=4.7, $p<.002$), serious violence (OR=37.6, $p<.0001$), and drug dealing (OR=192.5, $p<.0001$).

Gangs. Involvement in youth gangs has been implicated as a factor in many homicides (e.g., Braga, 2008). The results suggested that those convicted of homicide were more likely to be involved in gangs than their controls (48%, compared to none of the controls; OR=11.8, $p<.0001$). All except one of those convicted for homicide reported that their gang was involved in gang fights with other gangs. However, of the 13 gang offenders who were convicted of homicide, none identified themselves as a leader or top person in a gang and none reported that they had a desire to move up the ranks within the gang. Those convicted of homicide who joined a gang reported

Table 7.3 Prevalence and frequency of drug use by convicted homicide offenders and controls

Prevalence	Convicted homicide offenders	Controls	Convicted vs. controls (OR)
% Alcohol use	77.8	81.5	0.8
% Legal drugs	11.1	0	1.9
% Marijuana use	88.9	33.3	15.8*
% Hard drug use	18.5	0	2.2*
Mean alcohol use (times)	433	142	7.4*
Mean marijuana use (times)	335	190	8.8*

Note: $*p < .05$

that they did so at an average age of 13.9 (SD = 1.4) and that their gangs varied in size from 5 to over 100 (mean = 33, SD = 28).

Drug Use. Table 7.3 shows that the prevalence of alcohol use in the past year, or in the year prior to arrest, was similar for offenders and controls, but those convicted of homicide were somewhat more likely to report having used legal drugs (prescription or nonprescription) although the numbers were small. The prevalence of the use of illegal drugs was significantly higher among those who were convicted of homicide: 89% of convicted males reported using marijuana compared to about one-third of the controls (OR = 15.8, $p < .0001$). Similarly, 19% of those convicted of homicide reported using hard drugs compared to none of the controls (OR = 2.2, $p < .004$).

Participants were also asked about the number of times that they had used alcohol or drugs in the past year or in the year before their arrest. Those convicted of homicide reported a higher frequency of alcohol use than the controls (OR = 7.4, $p < .0001$). Similarly, convicted males also reported higher levels of marijuana use than the controls (OR = 8.8, $p < .0001$).

Psychopathy. Psychopathy is a constellation of psychological and behavioral traits that have been linked to an increased likelihood of criminal, and especially violent, behavior (Harpur, Hakstian, & Hare, 1988). Psychopathy was assessed using the 12-item psychopathy checklist-screening version (PCL-SV) which measures the four facets that have been proposed to comprise psychopathy, each on a 3-item scale. Higher scores reflect greater similarity to the prototypical psychopath. Facet 1 assesses the psychological characteristics of arrogance and deceitfulness; Facet 2 assesses deficient affective experience (e.g., lack of empathy and guilt); Facet 3 assesses an impulsive and irresponsible lifestyle; and Facet 4 assesses juvenile delinquency and criminal versatility.

Table 7.4 shows the means on the four factor scores of psychopathy and on the total score. Given that the cut-off point for the diagnosis of psychopathy is 18 (Hart, Cox, & Hare, 1995), and the average score of those convicted of homicide is 19, many of the homicide offenders would be considered psychopaths. When compared to their controls, those convicted of homicide scored significantly higher on all four PCL-SV facets and on the total score. The results show that two-thirds (18 of the 27) of homicide offenders scored 18 or higher on psychopathy, and therefore were

Table 7.4 Homicide offenders and controls: scores on the psychopathy checklist-screening version

	Convicted homicide offenders (mean)	Controls (mean)	Convicted vs. controls (OR)
Facet 1 (arrogance and deceitfulness)	3.5	1.9	3.8*
Facet 2 (deficient affective experience)	4.7	1.2	26.2*
Facet 3 (impulsive and irresponsible lifestyle)	5.5	2.2	54.1*
Facet 4 (juvenile delinquency and criminal versatility)	5.3	1.2	77.7*
Total	18.9	6.5	37.6*
Psychopath	66.7%	14.8%	11.5*

Note: *$p < .05$

putative psychopaths, compared with 4 out of the 27 homicide controls (14.8%; OR = 11.5; $p < .0001$). However, while the convicted males had a significantly higher total score, this was mainly driven by their higher scores on Facets 3 and 4. These factors comprise the more behavioral components of psychopathy. Differences were less on the more personality components (Facets 1 and 2).

Situational Factors

One of the great advantages of the interviews was to obtain information about situational factors proximal to the homicide. All those convicted of homicide were asked a set of questions about the situation in which their alleged homicide offense had occurred. Not all offenders responded to all questions and six of those convicted of homicide asserted that they had not committed the alleged offense. In these instances, the individuals were asked to describe what the police had stated about their alleged homicide offense. This information was also supplemented by the official police reports where these were available.

Reason for the Offense. The most common reasons given were a robbery gone badly (29%), that they were the victim of a robbery and acted in self-defense (25%), or that it was an argument that got out of hand (29%). Less common reasons mentioned drug deals (8%), gang victimization (4%), and a vehicle accident (4%). In a few cases, a robbery gone badly concerned the robbery of a drug dealer, and acting in self-defense concerned persons trying to steal drugs from the participant, so the reason for the offense was connected with drug use in more cases than was immediately apparent.

Offense Setting. The street was the most common setting for the homicide offenses (63%). Only 19% of offenses of those convicted of homicide occurred in the house of the victim.

Time of the Offense. A slightly higher number of the homicide offenses were committed either in the evening (35%; 7 p.m.–12 a.m.) or early morning (35%; 12 a.m.–6 a.m.) compared to the daylight hours (31%; 6 a.m.–6 p.m.).

Type of Weapon Used. The most common weapon used was a gun (77%). Only half of the guns belonged to the offenders. In most of the other cases, the guns belonged to the victim. Knives were used in two homicides, and a car was used in one homicide. The remainder of the weapons appeared to be weapons of convenience (a hammer, a phone cord, and a brick).

Co-offenders. When asked whether they had been alone or with others at the time the offense was committed, most of those convicted of homicide said that they were with others (66%).

Drug and Alcohol Use. Slightly less than half of the convicted males (45%) reported having consumed alcohol before the offense. Approximately 68% of those convicted of homicide reported having used drugs prior to the homicide. In all except one case, this drug was marijuana.

Knowledge of the Victim. The convicted males usually knew the victim before the offense (77%). When asked to report how they felt about the victim before the crime, most of the convicted males reported feeling indifferent about the victim (77%), while 12% disliked the victim and 12% liked the victim.

Feelings During the Commission of the Crime. The men were asked about the emotions that they had felt during the commission of the offense. The most common responses were feeling nothing (30%) or feeling scared (30%). The remainder of those convicted of homicide reported feeling angry (20%), sad or upset (15%), or satisfied (5%).

Behavior Immediately After the Offense. Immediately after the offense almost all of those convicted of homicide reported that they fled the scene (95%).

Feelings After the Offense. After the offense was committed, those convicted of homicide mostly reported that they felt nothing or felt numb (42%), while 32% said that they felt scared and 26% said that they felt sad or upset.

Conclusions

This chapter reported on the postevent interviews with convicted homicide offenders and their controls. We are convinced that there is merit in attempting to discover factors that are proximally related to the commission of a homicide. Perhaps in future research we will be able to link the long-term antisocial factors that have been uncovered by Farrington, Ttofi, and Coid (2009) and Loeber et al. (2005a) to the more immediate situational factors that have been identified in this chapter.

The interview results are concordant with findings in Chap. 3. The homicide offenders were much more extreme compared to the controls in almost all forms of problem behavior, and this was true for moderate and serious theft, serious violence, and drug dealing. The homicide offenders, with the exception of the use of alcohol and the use of legal drugs, also scored higher than the controls on all measures of drug consumption, including marijuana and hard drug use, and the frequency of alcohol and marijuana use. The homicide offenders also scored higher on all the facets of psychopathy (discussed more in detail in Chap. 10) and on engaging in gang activities. Two-thirds of the homicide offenders had PCL-SV scores that indicated that they were psychopaths, but this was less clear from their personality profile.

It should be noted that the demographics showed that none of the homicide offenders were married, and not surprisingly they tended to have fewer children. The overall impression is that homicide offenders have serious behavior problems, and it is probable that these problems make them less than suitable candidates for marriage and contribute to their social isolation. This also means that the possible reforming influence of a partner is less often available for the homicide offenders.

Chapter 8
Modeling the Impact of Preventive Interventions on the National Homicide Rate

Beth E. Ebel, Frederick P. Rivara, Rolf Loeber, and Dustin A. Pardini

One of the responses to the National Institute of Health's *State of the Science Report on Violence Prevention* in 2004 stated that "The practice of public policy in youth violence prevention is out of step with scientific evidence and leads to inefficient spending, failure to bring effective programs to youth, and adverse effects on children by supporting harmful programs" (cited in Tuma, Loeber, & Lochman, 2006, p. 455). The key question of how public policy can be better brought in line with evidence is particularly relevant to the putative effects of interventions on the wellbeing of populations, including the reduction of homicide.

Whereas the preceding chapters used longitudinal and cross-sectional/retrospective data to illustrate the development and prediction of homicide offending and homicide victimization, we now turn to the societal response to homicide. We are particularly interested in whether it is possible to prevent homicide offending (this chapter and Chap. 9), homicide victimization, and violence (reviewed in Chap. 9), and to estimate the benefits of intervention programs. This effort to prevent delinquency and violence contrasts with the prevailing response to crime by means of incarceration.

As demonstrated in this volume and in past studies, a great deal of research over the last few decades has shown that the origins of violence are found in childhood and adolescence. Very few violent offenders have a history free of youth behavioral problems (Farrington, 1996; Farrington & Loeber, 2000; Loeber & Farrington, 2000a; Loeber & Stouthamer-Loeber, 1998). Recent work on trajectories of aggression indicates that children begin to show physical aggression as infants, and that this peaks in the preschool years and then decreases throughout childhood and adolescence in most individuals (Tremblay et al., 2004). However, there is a group of children who do not learn to control this aggression, and nearly all of the later violent offenders come from this group (Broidy et al., 2003; Loeber et al., 2005b; Tremblay et al., 2004). Continuity in aggressive behavior over time is the hallmark of most violent offenders.

Because of this continuity of behavior, many investigators have turned their attention to developing and testing interventions to prevent violence by altering the

R. Loeber and D.P. Farrington, *Young Homicide Offenders and Victims,*
Longitudinal Research in the Social and Behavioral Sciences: An Interdisciplinary Series,
DOI 10.1007/978-1-4419-9949-8_8, © Springer Science+Business Media, LLC 2011

early life course, thereby preventing violence downstream (Welsh & Farrington, 2010). Interventions such as nurse home visiting (Olds et al., 1998), parent training (e.g., Webster-Stratton et al., 2001), early childhood education (Catalano, Arthur, Hawkins, Berglund, & Olson, 1998), and intensive programs for troubled youth (Borduin et al., 1995) have had both immediate and long-term effects. However, no attempt has been made to date to examine the potential impact of these interventions on fatal violence.

Typically, the efficacy of interventions to reduce or prevent offending is pursued through a comparison between an experimental and a control group, with the experimental group being exposed to a systematic intervention and the control group receiving either no intervention or an intervention as usual. In the best of evaluation studies, assignment of participants is done randomly to either the experimental or control groups (e.g., Campbell & Stanley, 1966; Committee on Improving Evaluation of Anti-Crime Programs, 2005). The latter, called randomized trials, can be contrasted with quasi-experimental interventions in which, for example, participants in the experimental group are matched to participants in the control group. Either way, criminologists often think that these are the only two ways in which evaluations of interventions can be accomplished, and have discounted the possibilities of using nonexperimental survey data for the purposes of evaluations.

An innovative aspect of this chapter and Chap. 9 is to use nonexperimental longitudinal data to model or simulate the impact of interventions. Simulation can be compared with asking the question "What if..." we changed one aspect of the data set, what impact would that have on future offending such as homicide? We propose that criminology can extend its scope, including the evaluation of interventions, by modeling such interventions on existing nonexperimental data, preferably longitudinal data with multiple measurements. Thus, along with modelers in other areas of science, such as aeronautics, weather forecasting, archeology, and economic forecasting (e.g., Epstein, 2006), we propose two lines of nonexperimental evaluations of interventions. Parameter estimation will be used to demonstrate the benefits of a nationwide intervention to reduce homicide offending (this chapter). In the second example, presented in Chap. 9, we will demonstrate that by using the PYS data, it is possible to simulate or model the efficacy to screen for high-risk individuals and then to apply a treatment that "knocks out" youth who otherwise would have been at risk of displaying violence, including homicide, or would have been at risk of becoming a victim of violence. In summary, in both chapters, we will use nonexperimental methods to demonstrate the benefits of interventions. We argue that simulation of interventions on rich longitudinal data, as available in the Pittsburgh Youth Study, has several advantages:

1. Tracking the impact of interventions over much longer periods of time than is usually available from relatively brief follow-ups after a randomized or quasi-experimental intervention.
2. The simulation can take advantage of the correlated structures of predictors and outcomes as recorded in the longitudinal data and examine the extent to which changes in one affect changes in the other.

3. The simulation can "knock-out" a percentage of the at-risk population and trace the impact of the knock-out on several outcomes over time, particularly changes in the homicide rate at the national level.

The main questions addressed in the current chapter are:

- When modeling nationwide interventions focused on high-risk youth, how much decrease in the national homicide rate can we expect?
- Is early intervention more efficient than later intervention?

The Impact of Early Interventions on a National Scale on the National Homicide Rate

Methods

The strategy in our modeling was to determine the baseline number of homicide deaths and resulting years of potential life lost (YPLL) due to violence by the cohort of males aged 18 in 2000. We then calculated the prevalence of violence in the cohort that would be expected if the selected interventions were implemented on a national scale, and the consequent change in the number of homicides as a result. We were interested in homicides committed by this cohort at any time during their life course. We only included males in the cohort because 90% of all homicide offenders in the USA are male (Fox & Zawitz, 2001), most of the longitudinal studies on delinquency and violence prevention programs have only included males, and the linkages between female childhood physical aggression and later violent offending are less clear (Broidy et al., 2003; Loeber et al., 1998a). While most interventions have targeted families or youths in urban environments and 91% of murders occur in urban neighborhoods (Fox & Zawitz, 2001), the essential elements of each intervention are applicable to urban and rural populations and therefore we did not confine our analysis only to urban males. We did not stratify by race because intervention effectiveness was generally not available stratified by race, and because we were modeling at the population level. The University of Washington institutional review board approved all study procedures.

Data Sources

Table 8.1 summarizes the data used in our models. The probability of incarceration for violent crimes was based on individuals committing an index crime. The number of homicides in the USA that would be committed by the cohort throughout their lives was estimated using age-specific homicide offending rates in 2000. The years lost due to homicide were calculated by subtracting the average age at death

Table 8.1 Variables used in violence prevention decision model

Variable	Value	Reference
Probability of being arrested if committed rape, robbery, or assault	0.256	Farrington, Langan, & Tonry (2004)
Probability of being incarcerated if convicted of rape, robbery, or assault	0.663	Farrington et al. (2004)
Probability of being incarcerated if committed murder	0.524	Farrington et al. (2004)
Life expectancy of US male at 25 years of age, 2001	75.9 years	CDC (Arias, Anderson, Kung, Murphy, & Kochanek, 2003)
Life expectancy of US female at 25 years of age, 2001	80.7 years	CDC (Arias et al., 2003)
Average age of homicide victim	25 years	CDC (Centers for Disease Control & Prevention, 2006)
Probability of male being violent by age 18	0.614	Pittsburgh Youth Study
Probability of arrest by age 18 if violent	0.397	Pittsburgh Youth Study
Probability of conviction for violent crime by age 25 if previously violent	0.321	Pittsburgh Youth Study
Probability of conviction for murder by age 25 if previously violent by age 18	0.024	Pittsburgh Youth Study
Probability of previously violent by age 18 if murderer by age 25	1.0	Pittsburgh Youth Study
Mean incarceration length for murder	126.2 months	Farrington et al. (2004)
Mean incarceration length for rape, robbery, assault	33.0 months	Farrington et al. (2004)
Mean annual prison cost per inmate, US$ 2002	$23,194 (Range $ 8,128 Arkansas, $44,379 Maine)	Stephan (Stephan, 2004) ($22,650 in 2001, inflated using CPI-U index from BLS)
Murder victims, US 2002	14,054	Federal Bureau of Investigation (2003)
Estimated murders committed by males, 2002	12,691	Federal Bureau of Investigation (2003)
Ratio of victims/persons convicted of homicide, 2002	0.889	Federal Bureau of Investigation (2003)
Proportion of murder victims who were male, 2002	77%	Federal Bureau of Investigation (2003)
Percentage of convicted murderers who are male, 2002	90.3%	Federal Bureau of Investigation (2003)
Total number of US murderers, 2002	15,813	Federal Bureau of Investigation (2003)

(continued)

Table 8.1 (continued)

Variable	Value	Reference
Discount rate applied to years of potential life lost for murder victims and years of incarceration for murderers	3%	Siegel, Weinstein, Russell & Gold (1996)
Discount factor for effectiveness of model programs when implemented in practice	50%	Estimate based on data from Lipsey, documenting that program effectiveness for demonstration programs was between 44 and 56% less than programs replicated in practice (Lipsey, 2003).
Intervention participation rates	20%	Olds nurse home visitation project (Olds et al., 1998)
	30%	Perry preschool project. Participation rate estimated from implementation of Perry model in Georgia
	21.5%	Multisystemic therapy (Schaeffer & Borduin, 2005)

from homicide in 2000 (25 years) from the average US life expectancy of a US male (75.9 years) and a US female (80.7 years) at age 25, weighted by their relative representation among victims of murder. The years lost due to incarceration were determined by summing the average sentence time served for homicide and other violent crimes. Incarceration costs were derived by multiplying average sentence time served by the annual cost of incarceration. A 3% discount rate for both costs and years of potential life saved was used in all analyses, reflecting the fact that saving costs or lives is valued more highly in the present than in the future (Weinstein, Siegel, Gold, Kamlet, & Russell, 1996).

No intervention studies have examined a large enough sample or followed participants long enough to determine the number of homicides that were prevented through the intervention. Our model was based on determining the proportion of individuals who received the intervention and were subsequently not involved with violence compared to the proportion who were involved with violence in the absence of the intervention. This model was then applied to the proportion of homicide offenders in the cohort who had a prior history of violence and thus might have been affected by the intervention.

Among the 506 boys in the oldest cohort, 12 were convicted of homicide by age 25. Among the 503 boys in the youngest cohort, ten were convicted of homicide. Each of these 22 murderers had violent behavior before age 18: all had either self-reported violence or arrests for violence before age 18, and all had previously been arrested and convicted of a violent offense. We did not include the middle cohort because these boys were not followed for the same prolonged longitudinal period.

Earlier studies tend to have extremely limited data on the prior violent histories of individuals who committed murder after the age of 25. Studies based on official records are limited by the availability of juvenile justice data, which are usually kept separately from adult criminal records, as well as by the absence of self-reported data on violent behavior. We therefore used the same proportion (i.e., 1.0) of homicide offenders with violent behavior before age 18 for individuals who murdered after age 25 as for those who murdered before age 25. The ratio of victims to murderers was based on US data for 2002 (Farrington, Langan, & Tonry, 2004). The mean annual cost of incarceration was $23,194 but ranged from a low of $8,128 in Arkansas to a high of $44,379 in Maine. Estimates for time incarcerated were derived from published data on time served for homicide (Farrington et al., 2004).

Interventions During Childhood and Adolescence

We undertook focused reviews of the literature and contacted experts in the field of violence prevention to determine effective interventions to decrease the prevalence of violent offending. Databases searched include Medline, the Cochrane Library, PsycInfo, ERIC, EconLit, CINAHL, the National Criminal Justice Reference Service (NCJRS), and the RAND Promising Practices Network. Each of the above databases was searched for randomized controlled trials, meta-analyses, and systematic reviews concerning violence prevention in youth. Some of the interventions found in the literature search were designed to reach the general population or younger "high-risk" children (home visiting, early childhood education, school-based programs, and parent education). Others were targeted at delinquent youth (family therapy, multisystemic therapy, therapeutic foster care). Separate tailored searches were then performed for each of these intervention categories to detect additional studies. The bibliographies of included articles and relevant review articles were searched for additional material, and we contacted experts in the field with the aim of including every relevant violence prevention intervention among youths.

To be included, we required that interventions report longitudinal follow-up data into adulthood, and that changes in subsequent arrest or violent arrest rates be measured relative to a control group. We included interventions with arrest outcomes as measured by official police or court records rather than self-reported violent behavior or arrests. We considered interventions for three time periods: early childhood, school age, and adolescence.

Nurse home visiting beginning during the prenatal period and extending into early infancy and childhood has been examined with randomized controlled trials. Olds and his colleagues have followed an initial intervention and control cohort of 400 families to age 15, and have shown that the incidence of arrests was reduced by 54% among children whose mothers had received nurse visitations during pregnancy and infancy, compared to control children (17% in the visitation group compared to 36% in the control group) (Olds et al., 1998). Intervention children also had a lower incidence of convictions and probation violations (10% vs. 27%).

There have been a number of studies demonstrating the effect of early childhood education on later delinquency and violence. The longest duration longitudinal study of early childhood education is the Perry Preschool Project in which individuals have been followed to age 40 (Schweinhart et al., 2005). This was an intervention at ages 3 and 4 for high-risk inner city youth, and it was evaluated using a randomized trial design. The arrest rate for violence by age 40 in the experimental group compared to the control group was reduced by 33%. As there is evidence that research/demonstration programs may be less effective when replication is attempted on a larger scale under real-life conditions, we assumed that interventions were 50% less effective when replicated on a larger scale (Table 8.1), basing this estimate on the available literature (Lipsey, 2003).

A number of investigators have conducted studies of school-based intervention programs for high-risk youth (Catalano et al., 1998). These programs have shown a variety of important positive effects including decreasing aggression and improving prosocial behavior. One successful program is the Seattle Social Development Project (Hawkins, Catalano, Kosterman, Abbott, & Hill, 1999). This found reductions in subsequent arrest as a consequence of the school-based violence prevention program among students followed from grade 1 to age 18, although results did not reach statistical significance (RR = 0.76, 95% CI 0.50, 1.14). A later study followed participants to 21 years of age (Hawkins et al., 2005). While there were lasting effects on school performance, emotional and mental health, there was no longer a difference between the full intervention group and the control group in the incidence of arrest (12% vs. 10%, $p = .61$) nor in the report of any crime in the past year (29% vs. 28%, $p = 0.87$). A study by Tremblay and colleagues found a reduction in self-reported juvenile delinquency but did not find a significant reduction in arrests over the duration of the study period (Tremblay et al., 1995).

Successful interventions for adolescents who have been involved with violence include therapeutic foster care and multisystemic treatment. One program presented data on the long-term reduction of violent arrests following multisystemic treatment. Four years postintervention, there was a 63% reduction in subsequent violent arrests for juvenile delinquents in the program (Borduin et al., 1995). Since studies of therapeutic foster care had shorter follow-ups, we elected to model the effect of multisystemic therapy on subsequent homicides.

No studies have examined multiple interventions applied to the same population. We chose to model three effective interventions which reach children at different stages of their development. Each was chosen because it was a randomized controlled trial, reported long-term follow-up rates, and measured subsequent arrests or arrests for violent crime (Table 8.2). The Olds Nurse Home Visitation Project model addresses families around the birth of the child and in infancy. The Perry Preschool Project model provides early childhood education to families at risk. Our literature review and consultation with experts found no middle school intervention with long-term effectiveness on documented arrest rates. The multisystemic therapy (MST) model works with adolescent offenders who have already shown evidence of delinquency.

Table 8.2 Interventions before age 18 to prevent later violence

Intervention/source	Variable	Estimate (range)	Age period	Outcome measure, intervention vs. control group
Olds nurse home visitation project (Olds et al., 1998)	Reduction of incidence of arrest	RR = 0.54 (0.31, 0.68)	Intervene with family during pregnancy and infancy	Comparison of control group to group receiving nurse visits during pregnancy and infancy. 29/176 (intervention) vs. 53/148 (control) had been arrested in 15-year follow-up period (16.5% vs. 35.8%)
Perry preschool project (Schweinhart et al., 2005)	Reduction of subsequent violent arrest	RR = 0.67 (0.44, 1.08)	Early Childhood	Proportion with violent arrests: 0.32 (intervention) vs. 0.48 (control), $p = .09$, $n_i = 58$, $n_c = 65$ at enrollment
Multisystemic therapy (Schaeffer & Borduin, 2005)	Reduction of subsequent violent arrests after follow-up to mean age 28.8 years (13.7 years of follow-up)	RR = 0.48 (0.26, 0.85)	Adolescence	Proportion with violent arrests: 0.141 (13/92 in intervention group) vs. 0.298 (25/84 in control group)

Note: RR = Relative Risk

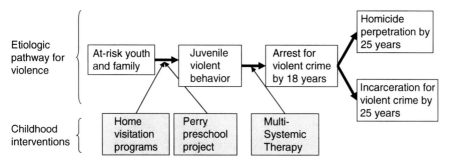

Fig. 8.1 Violence intervention model for decision analysis, violence prevention interventions in childhood and adolescence

Decision Analysis

A decision analysis tree was used to determine the impact of each intervention scenario on baseline deaths due to homicide, years of potential life lost due to homicide, and cost of incarceration (Fig. 8.1). These interventions were chosen because they represent model interventions that could be replicated on a larger scale. The first three scenarios separately measured the impact of three interventions outlined in Table 8.2. The fourth scenario measured the potential impact if all three interventions were implemented with cumulative results, i.e., a home visitation program and school-based intervention would reduce violent behaviors and subsequent juvenile delinquency. Among the resulting males with delinquent behavior, we assumed that a multisystemic therapy intervention would reduce subsequent violent arrests.

The decision analysis models were constructed using Data™ 4.0 (TreeAge Software, Inc., Williamstown, MA). The model estimated the number of homicides committed by a cohort of 18-year-olds, incorporating the one-time effect of interventions on violence. This cohort was followed as members aged, and estimates for homicides, victim years of potential life lost (YPLL) due to homicide and incarceration cost were calculated. Sensitivity testing was performed for the critical variables used in the model to explore the potential impact on homicides, YPLL, and incarceration costs using the ranges determined from previous studies or derived as discussed above. For the cumulative intervention model, a sensitivity analysis was conducted using Monte Carlo methods in which key parameters were varied simultaneously, performed with Data 4.0™ (TreeAge Software, Inc., Williamstown, MA). Distributions were sampled 10,000 times for the final analysis.

Recognizing that intervention programs conducted under "real-life" conditions are unlikely to achieve the results measured under more rigorous study conditions, we assumed that program effectiveness for each intervention was 50% less in the replication than in the original test of the program (Lipsey, 2003). Finally, not all families will wish to participate in an intervention. We used participation rates for each intervention program from the literature to determine the proportion of families willing to participate (Table 8.1).

Results

The Pittsburgh Youth Study provided longitudinal data to construct a model of the evolution of violent behavior among 1,009 urban males in the oldest and youngest cohorts followed from childhood until 25 years of age (see Table 2.1 in Chap. 2). The majority of males (61%) reported violent behavior in their youth, although only a small fraction (2.4%) went on to commit and be convicted of murder. No murders were committed by males without a history of violent behavior. Even among those who reported violent behaviors, no subsequent murders were committed by males without a prior conviction for violence before 25 years of age. Excluding nonnegligent manslaughter, an estimated 14,054 US individuals were victims of homicide in 2002, and we estimated that 12,691 were killed by male perpetrators.

Early home visitation programs with at-risk families could potentially prevent 21.7% (95% CI 4.1%, 33.8%) of all US homicides annually, with 52,180 years of potential life saved annually. Such programs have the potential to reduce incarceration costs by $3.5 billion ($0.7–$5.5 billion).

An early childhood education program similar to the Perry Preschool Program could potentially reduce subsequent murders by up to 24% (95% CI −5.3 to 39%), saving an estimated 3,044 lives annually, and resulting in $3.9 billion savings in incarceration costs (Table 8.3), although the confidence intervals around these estimates are large. National implementation of multisystemic therapy for juvenile delinquents with prior arrests could reduce homicide rates by 6.1% annually (95% CI −3.1 to 11.3%), resulting in $789 million savings in incarceration costs.

Each of these three types of programs targets a different stage of childhood, and their effects could potentially be combined to reduce violent behavior and its consequences, although this has not been tried in practice. We evaluated the cumulative impact of three simultaneous interventions (nurse home visiting, early childhood education for families at risk, and multisystemic therapy), and then estimated confidence intervals assuming a three-way sensitivity analysis in which each intervention was allowed to vary from least to most effective simultaneously. This model found that the combination of these interventions in childhood or adolescence could potentially reduce 33% (95% CI −2.0 to 62.2%) of all murders, saving 4,205 lives annually and resulting in $5.2 billion (95% CI $−0.68 billion to $10.4 billion) lifetime savings in incarceration costs alone (Table 8.3).

Table 8.3 Impact of childhood and adolescent interventions on reduction of homicide by urban males, years of potential life saved, and years of life incarcerated, and cost savings due to reduced incarceration, United States 2002

Intervention scenario	Percent reduction in number of murders	Estimated lives saved with intervention	Discounted years of potential life saved	Discounted reduction in years of incarceration	Cost savings from reduction in years of incarceration ($US millions, 2002)
Olds nurse home visitation project	21.7%	2,760	52,180	151,305	$3,510
	(4.1%, 33.8%)	(526, 4,290)	(9,950, 81,117)	(29,869, 235,022)	($693, $5,451)
Perry preschool project	24.0%	3,044	57,557	166,833	$3,870
	(−5.3%, 39.2%)	(−675, 4,989)	(−12,767, 94,329)	(−37,042, 273,537)	($−859, $6,344)
Multisystemic therapy with juvenile delinquents	6.1%	771	14,579	34,036	$789
	(−3.1%, 11.3%)	(−391, 1,440)	(−7,394, 27,221)	(−16,737, 62,983)	($−388, $1,461)
Cumulative impact of early childhood, school-based, and MST programs	33%	4,205	79,496	223,472	$5,183
	(−2.0%, 62.2%)	(−258, 10,561)	(−4,886, 199,686)	(−29,319, 448,677)	($−680, $10,407)

Notes: Program effectiveness was estimated at 50% of study values at national scale

Numbers in parentheses refer to a range of values based on sensitivity analyses

Conclusions

In 1993, McGinnis and Foege (1993) recast the discussion of causes of death by emphasizing the behavioral contributions to mortality, and their estimates were updated in 2004 (Mokdad, Marks, Stroup, & Gerberding, 2004). Their work pointed the way to re-examination of potential preventive strategies for modifying behavioral risk factors. As is the case with smoking (Rivara et al., 2004) and harmful drinking (McCarty et al., 2004), the antecedents of violent behavior also begin in childhood. This conclusion is in line with results from prospective studies of juveniles at risk for delinquency (Loeber & Farrington, 2000) and homicidal behavior (Loeber et al., 2005). Further, as shown in Chaps. 4 and 5, youths who commit violent crimes have a high probability of becoming adult violent offenders. A recent study examined the criminal histories of men who were executed in Texas in 1997 for murder, finding that 86.5% had a juvenile criminal history (van Soest, Park, Johnson, & McPhail, 2003). Thus, there is strong evidence that continuity of antisocial behavior is a hallmark of future homicide offenders. That continuity also offers ample opportunities to intervene.

This chapter examined three intervention strategies with promise for changing the developmental trajectory leading from violent behaviors in childhood to delinquency, violent crime, and murder. If implemented on a national scale, nurse home visiting programs, early childhood education programs, and multisystemic therapy with juvenile delinquents all hold promise for reducing lives lost to homicide by 33%, saving an estimated 4,205 lives annually, 79,070 years of potential life lost, and up to $5.1 billion in the cost of incarcerating violent criminals.

The effectiveness of the three interventions studied here may represent a "best case scenario," and lower effectiveness might be found if such programs were implemented on a wider scale. We have attempted to adjust for real-life conditions by assuming that model programs would only be half as effective when implemented on a larger scale (Barnoski, 2004; Lipsey, 2003). While most assumptions are cost savings, it should be noted that if "worst case" assumptions held, there might not be program benefits (Table 8.3), highlighting that we have imprecise estimates of program impact with wide confidence intervals. Finally, we have provided estimates of program effectiveness for three model interventions separately, and then attempted to estimate the combined effectiveness if all three interventions were implemented together, using confidence intervals based on the literature. It is unknown whether these interventions would, in fact, have a fully multiplicative effect, or whether there is a group of youths who would be recalcitrant to interventions at all levels, reducing the overall impact.

While recent trends toward decreasing levels of violence in the USA are encouraging, violent crime results in enormous social and economic costs. In 2002, there were 14,054 murders (Federal Bureau of Investigation, 2003), resulting in 235,000 years of potential life lost, discounted over time. In fiscal year 2001, Federal, State and local governments spent over $167 billion for police protection, corrections, and judicial and legal activities (Bureau of Justice Statistics, 2004a).

Criminal activities result in economic losses of $15.5 billion annually (Bureau of Justice Statistics, 2004b). There are significant costs to the victims of violent crime and their families, including the loss of life, economic support, companionship, and security.

There is a growing body of research on the prevention and treatment of violence, with increasing importance given to carefully conducted, randomized experiments (Farrington & Welsh, 2006). Researchers have attempted to estimate the benefits and costs of prevention and early intervention programs, finding that proven programs for juvenile offending, home visitation for high-risk mothers, early childhood education, and the Seattle Social Development Project resulted in net benefits per participant ranging from $1,900 to $17,200 (Aos, Lieb, Mayfield, Miller, & Pennucci, 2004). Such results highlight the preventable nature of violent behavior and the potential reductions in violent crime, homicide, jail time, and economic costs as a result of diverting children and adolescents from the trajectory of escalating violent behaviors.

Chapter 9
Modeling the Impact of Interventions on Local Indicators of Offending, Victimization, and Incarceration

Rolf Loeber and Rebecca Stallings

In Chap. 8 we laid out the rationale behind simulation (modeling) studies to ascertain the impact of interventions on reducing violence, particularly the national homicide rates in a cohort of males aged 18 in 2000. The interventions considered were nurse home visiting, a preschool intellectual enrichment program, and multisystemic therapy. In contrast with Chap. 8 that dealt with the impact of preventive interventions on the national homicide rate, this chapter deals with the impact of preventive and remedial interventions on local indicators of offending and victimization in the PYS (homicide offenders, homicide victims, arrests for violence, serious delinquency, and incarceration of offenders). The main questions are as follows:

- To what extent does an intervention with a success rate of 30% that focuses on high-risk boys at a young age (ages 7–13; Screen 1) reduce arrests for violence as shown in the age–crime curve, and other indicators of violent offending and incarceration?

The next questions concern whether an early intervention is better than a later intervention:

- Does an intervention at age 14 only based on arrest for violence have sufficient benefits if an intervention already has taken place at an earlier age?
- What is the yield of an intervention at age 14 based on arrest for violence without an intervention at an earlier age?
- How well do the two interventions compare when serious delinquency is the outcome?
- Does an intervention at a young age have a higher yield in reducing the frequency of serious delinquency than an intervention at age 13?

In prior chapters we examined predictors and precursors to violence, homicide offenders, and homicide victims (Chaps. 4–7). Here we concentrate on two indicators, a high-risk score at screening (ages 7–13) and arrest for violence (by age 14), because each can be incorporated in a screening device to identify those who could

R. Loeber and D.P. Farrington, *Young Homicide Offenders and Victims*,
Longitudinal Research in the Social and Behavioral Sciences: An Interdisciplinary Series,
DOI 10.1007/978-1-4419-9949-8_9, © Springer Science+Business Media, LLC 2011

benefit from an intervention to reduce future violence. Thus, we will consider for this chapter two categories of risk groups of youth that are most relevant: first, those youth who score high on an index of disruptive/delinquent behavior early in life, i.e., at the first assessment of the PYS (see below for details). The second category of individuals consists of those arrested for violence by age 14 (i.e., robbery or simple or aggravated assault).

Availability of longitudinal follow-up data allows the modeling of the impact of interventions on a variety of outcomes at different ages. Key among these outcomes is the universally observed age–crime curve showing an increase in offending starting in early adolescence, a peaking in mid- to late-adolescence, and a subsequent decrease in a offending (Farrington, 1986). We focus on the age–crime curve instead of prevalence in a given year because the age–crime curve provides more information about the development of offending for a population of youth, and the presence (or reoccurrence) of offenders across many years rather than in a few years of follow-up, which is typical for the evaluation of most interventions. In addition, our emphasis on the age–crime curve is based on the assumption that: (a) community crime levels are the result of the accumulation and part-overlap between successive age–crime curves of successive birth cohorts, and that (b) changes in community crime levels are dependent on increases (or decreases) in the age–crime curves of successive birth cohorts.

Although the age–crime curve is similar in many studies, its shape can vary from one birth cohort to another, with some age–crime curves being higher and broader than other age–crime curves (e.g., Loeber, Farrington, Stouthamer-Loeber, & White 2008; Fabio, Cohen, & Loeber, in press), indicating that violence goes on longer and that the proportion of new cases is larger than in other birth cohorts. It is important to examine whether interventions have a larger impact on a high and broad age–crime curve compared to a lower and narrower age–crime curve. In addition, we are interested in to what extent two types of interventions reduce arrest for violence, homicide offenders, and homicide victims between adolescence and early adulthood.

We aim to model in the PYS (for study details, see Chap. 2) two types of screens and related interventions. The two screens were applied in sequence (see Fig. 9.1), but will also be assessed separately.

Screen 1 for Intervention 1. First, we are modeling an intervention that targets those boys who score high on a disruptive/delinquency index at the beginning of the study (detailed in Loeber et al., 1998). The choice of this risk score was governed by prior research, showing that early disruptive problems and early forms of delinquency are among the best predictors of later delinquency, violence and homicide (Farrington, 1991; Loeber & Dishion, 1983; Loeber & Farrington, 2001; Loeber et al., 2005a). Screen 1 was based on the screening risk score computed from data collected at the first assessment for each of the three cohorts at ages 7, 10, and 13, for the youngest, middle, and oldest cohorts, respectively (Loeber et al., 1998a; p. 35; $N = 256$ for the youngest cohort; $N = 259$ for middle cohort; and $N = 257$ for the oldest cohort).

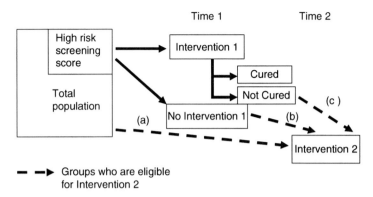

Fig. 9.1 Representation of the simulation of the sequence of the two interventions

Information included in this screen concerns the following behaviors: attack, run away, set fires, steal from other places than the home, truancy, vandalism, steal from car, robbery, steal bicycle, shoplift, steal car, weapon attack, gang fight, hit/hurt teacher, hit/hurt parent, joyride, burglary, arrested, liquor use, sniff glue, and marijuana use.[1] Whenever possible, the information was extracted from lifetime questions in addition to behavior which took place in the past half year. To strengthen the construct, three informants reported on the above behaviors: the youth, his parent, and his teacher. The high-risk score was a score of more than one antisocial behavior for the youngest cohort, a score of more than two for the middle cohort, and a score of more than three for the oldest cohort. Across the cohorts, there were 772 high-risk cases; 30% of these constitute 232 cases.

Screen 2 for Intervention 2. The second screen consists of arrest for violence (robbery, simple assault, or aggravated assault). Because the three cohorts differed in age at the beginning of the study, the time windows for arrest for violence were slightly different for each cohort: ages 9–19 for the youngest cohort; ages 10–22 for the middle cohort; and, ages 13–25 for the oldest cohort. The focus of Screen 2 were three categories of individuals, all of whom were arrested for violence by age 14, that is: (a) those remaining in the total population minus those with a high-risk screening score (Fig. 9.1a); (b) those from the high-risk screening score group who did not receive Intervention 1 (Fig. 9.1b); and (c) those from the high-risk screening group who received Intervention 1, but who were not "cured" (Fig. 9.1c). Out of these three groups, we assumed for the sake of modeling again a success rate of 30%.

---

[1]The exception was that aggressive problem behaviors from the youth's self-report were not included because of studies showing that children, compared to adults, are not always the best reporters on their own aggression (Loeber, Green, & Lahey, 1990; Loeber, Green, Lahey, & Stouthamer-Loeber, 1989).

Four court sources of arrest (charged for a crime) for violence were used for the juvenile and adult years. Juvenile court data were obtained from the Allegheny County Juvenile Court records for offenses within Allegheny County from the participants up to 2001 (data collection covered ages 10 through 18 for all three cohorts). In addition, the Pennsylvania Juvenile Court Judges' Commission provided data on all offenses by participants throughout Pennsylvania up to 1997 (data covered ages 10–16 for the youngest cohort and ages 10 through 18 for both the middle cohort and oldest cohorts). The Pennsylvania State Police Repository provided state criminal history record information through Spring 2001 (covering up to age 20 for the youngest cohort, up to age 23 for the middle cohort and up to age 26 for the oldest cohort). The Federal Bureau of Investigation provided federal criminal history record information in the Spring of 2001 (data covered ages 18–20 for the youngest, 18–23 for the middle, and 18–26 for the oldest cohort).

To obtain information about arrest for violence, each of the four types of records were searched and coded for offense date, offense category, and disposition, according to the format developed by Weinrott (1975) and further improved by Maguin, Zucker, & Fitzgerald (1994). In addition, we instituted an Official Records Project (ORP), consisting of a compilation and integration of youths' court records collected from Allegheny County, the Commonwealth of Pennsylvania, and the Federal Bureau of Investigation. The coding system followed the definitions of crimes in the FBI Uniform Crime Reports and corresponds with the format used by the National Center for Juvenile Justice.

We will consider two versions of a second screen:

(a) *Screen 2 After Screen 1.* Because we expect that the risk status of young boys is not fully evident at Time 1, and also because we expect that the first screen may not identify all at-risk youth, we will model a second screen consisting of arrest by the police for a violent act for those boys who were not successfully treated of an intervention after having been identified by means of Screen 1, and those boys whose violence emerged after Screen 1. As shown in Fig. 9.1, we modeled two interventions occurring in sequence with Screen 1 and Intervention 1 serving as a first "net," while Screen 2 and Intervention 2 served as a second "net" for those who remained in the potentially treatable category of individuals after intervention 1 (for details see Methods below).

The sequential application of the screens will allow us to model the degree to which a second intervention based on police arrest for violence (Screen 2) improves the yield of an early intervention based on Screen 1. In other words, what is the yield of intervening with youth at-risk at a young age before contact with the police, vs. intervening at a young age and following a police contact for violence?

(b) *Screen 2 Alone.* In the second version of Screen 2, we will model the realistic situation for many communities that youth are identified only through the justice system, in this case through arrest for violence. Thus, we would model the situation in which alternative screens at a young age (such as Screen 1) for a given community are not available and that Screen 2 through arrest for violence is the only option.

Modeling the Impact of Interventions

The interventions modeled after each screen are inspired by the best intervention programs (Lipsey & Wilson, 1998) evaluated by the comparison of an experimental sample receiving the intervention vs. a control sample not receiving the program (or receiving an alternative program). For the present modeling exercise, we modeled interventions in which the experimental group outperformed the control group by 30%, corresponding to a standardized mean different (d) effect size of .3. The justification for our level of treatment efficacy was as follows. Lipsey and Wilson in their meta-analysis of treatments (1998, p. 332) found that the most effective interventions had an effect size d of about .4. In order to be conservative, we adopted a treatment effect size d of .3, corresponding to a decrease of 30% in the number convicted when comparing the experimental to the control group.

The reason why $d = .3$ corresponds approximately to a 30% decrease in offenders is as follows. Lipsey and Wilson (2001) showed that, when there are equal numbers of persons in experimental and control groups, $d = 2r/\sqrt{1 - r^2}$. When $d = .3$, d is approximately $2r$. Farrington and Loeber (1989) showed that, in a 2×2 table, r was approximately equal to the difference in proportions.

Consider the following table:

	NO	O	T
Experimental	65	35	100
Control	50	50	100

Where O = no. of offenders, NO = no. of nonoffenders, T = total. In this table, the difference in proportions of offenders between the experimental group (.35) and the control group (.50) is .15, and $r = .15$ in this table. However, the decrease in the number of offenders is from 50 to 35, a 30% decrease. Therefore, a 30% decrease in the number of offenders corresponds approximately to $d = .3$. The approximation is somewhat worse with other assumptions (e.g., that the number in the experimental group is different from the number in the control group) but is good enough to justify our assumption that an effective intervention could reduce the number of offenders by about 30%.

The simulation research was done on longitudinal data from the PYS (Loeber et al., 1998, 2008) for the youngest, middle, and oldest cohorts. Details about the youngest, middle, and oldest cohorts can be found in Chap. 2. Since limited information was available on self-reported delinquency for the middle cohort, reports of incarceration and the best estimate of serious delinquency are not included in the results for that cohort.

We modeled two types of interventions, one at the beginning of the study (ages 7, 10, and 13 for the youngest, middle, and oldest cohorts, respectively), and a second intervention at age 14 for each of the cohorts. The modeling of each intervention consists of "knocking out" or eliminating a random sample of 30% from the individuals identified by each screen as at risk and examining the impact of the modeled intervention on subsequent delinquency outcomes for the whole population of young men.

In modeling the impact of interventions following the two screens, we focus on six delinquency outcomes:

Arrest for Violence. This construct uses data from the Official Records Project (Loeber et al., 2008, p. 41), a compilation of participants' court records collected from Allegheny County, the Commonwealth of Pennsylvania, and the Federal Bureau of Investigation. The construct represents whether the youth was arrested and charged with moderate violence (simple assault) or serious violence (robbery, aggravated assault, aggravated indecent assault, homicide, forcible rape, involuntary deviate sexual intercourse, and spousal sexual assault) by age 20 for the youngest cohort, age 24 for the middle cohort, and age 26 for the oldest cohort.

Homicide Offenders. Details about the homicide offenders and their homicide can be found in Chap. 2, this volume; all 37 homicide offenders are included in the simulation analyses.

Homicide Victims. Details about the homicide victims can be found in Chap. 3. All 39 homicide victims are included in the simulation analyses.

Incarceration. This is based on several sources of information on the number of weeks the participant spent in correctional facilities, including juvenile detention facilities.[2] Incarceration data were only available for the youngest and oldest cohorts.

All-Source Serious Offending. This construct combines the prevalence of serious violence and serious theft and was made using reported and official conviction data. Reported data combines information from the boys' self-reported delinquency and information about the boys' delinquency based on parent's and teacher's reports (see Loeber et al., 2008 for details).

Frequency of Delinquent Acts. An additional measure of the all-source serious offending consists of the frequency of serious offending per offender.

---

[2] Because the official records gave very inadequate information on the duration of incarceration, we made use of the following sources of information: At Wave A and Waves J–T, the caretaker reported incarcerations on the Family Health questionnaire. Beginning at Wave K for the oldest sample and Wave V for the youngest, the Subject Health questionnaire answered by the participant replaced Family Health and collected the same data about incarceration. Lifetime data on incarceration were also collected from the caretaker at Wave G. For the youngest sample at Waves L–T, the Caretaker Demographics questionnaire asked the reason for and duration of any separation from the caretaker, and incarcerations reported there were added to the construct. Beginning at Wave O for the oldest sample, the Subject Demographics questionnaire asked, "How would you describe the way you live now?"; if a participant described himself as incarcerated but the incarceration was not reported in any other questionnaire, the construct was set to missing because he had been incarcerated but we did not know the number of weeks. Beginning at Wave U for the oldest sample and Wave V for the youngest, that question specified whether the participant had been incarcerated all year or was incarcerated only at present; if all year, the construct was set to 52 weeks.

Results

Figure 9.2 shows the age–crime for arrest for violence in the three cohorts without the simulated interventions. Arrest for violence gradually increased from age 11, peaked around age 18 and then decreased with age 25 being the terminal point in the available data. In total, the graph represents almost two-and-half thousand arrests ($N = 2,415$) for violence for the 1,517 individuals in the study.

Question 1: *To what extent does an intervention with a success rate of 30% that focuses on high-risk boys at a young age (ages 7–13; Screen 1) reduce arrests for violence as shown in the age–crime curve, and other indicators of offending, and incarceration?* Figure 9.3 shows that the intervention lowered the age–crime curve for arrest for violence, especially after age 13. The intervention led to 484 fewer arrests for violence, constituting a reduction of 20.0%. Not shown in the age–crime curve is that the intervention also has the benefit of reducing the homicide offenders by a third (from 37 to 24, or 35.9%) and the homicide victims by almost a third (from 39 to 25, or 35.9%). In addition, the intervention led to a reduction in the weeks of incarceration from 24,810 to 17,546 weeks, which amounted to a reduction more than 6, 264 weeks or 29.3%. Translated in years, the intervention reduced incarceration by 120.5 years.[3]

Question 2: *Does an intervention at age 14 only based on arrest for violence have sufficient benefits if an intervention already has taken place at an earlier age?* As mentioned, it can be argued that an intervention program that just focuses on high-risk offenders at a young age is too narrow and that it makes more sense to add to it an intervention program that focuses on known violent youth as well. For the second intervention, we modeled a program that focused on violent offenders at age 14 for all three cohorts. We again set the success rate at 30% of the program, thus realizing that not all violent youth would be effectively helped.

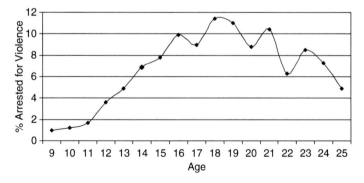

Fig. 9.2 Age–crime curve for percent arrested for violence without intervention (youngest, middle, and oldest cohorts)

---

[3]The incarceration data are based on the youngest and oldest cohorts only.

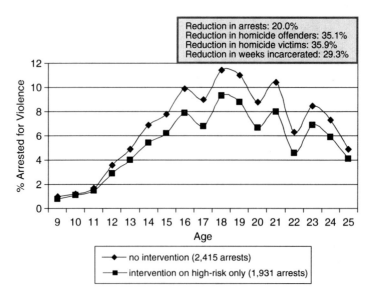

Fig. 9.3 Age–crime curves of percent arrested for violence before and after intervention on high-risk participants only (youngest, middle, and oldest cohorts)

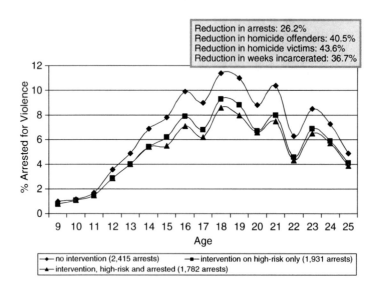

Fig. 9.4 Age–crime curves for percent arrested for violence before and after intervention on high-risk participants, followed by intervention on participants arrested by age 14 for robbery or assault (youngest, middle, and oldest cohorts)

Figure 9.4 shows that the implementation of Interventions 1 and 2 in sequence, compared to Intervention 1 only, further slightly lowered the age–crime curve, especially after age 14 (not surprisingly because that was the age of Intervention 2) and prior to age 20. Thus, the addition of Intervention 2 had no noticeable effect on the age–crime curve in young adulthood, ages 22–25. The reduction in arrests for violence for Interventions 1 and 2 in sequence consisted of 633 fewer arrests, which was 26.2% (from 2,415 to 1,782 arrests), thus only somewhat better than the effect of Intervention 1 alone (35.1%). More significantly, the combined interventions 1 and 2 produced a 43.6% reduction in homicide offenses, which was substantially better than intervention 1 alone (35.9%). In contrast, adding Intervention 2 to Intervention 1 only marginally improved the reduction in homicide victims (43.6% compared to 35.9%). Finally, Fig. 9.4 shows that the implementation of interventions 1 and 2 in sequence substantially reduced the number of weeks of incarceration from 29.2% for Intervention 1 only compared to 36.7% for Interventions 1 and 2.[4]

In summary, the first intervention with at-risk boys at a young age would have substantial benefits in reducing about one-third of all homicide offenders and one-third of the homicide victims. In addition, the first intervention would lead to a substantial reduction in the burden for the justice system, with a one fifth reduction in arrests for violence and a fifth reduction in weeks of incarceration. The average cost figure of incarceration mentioned in Chap. 8 of $23,194 per year per offender, means that the first intervention would lead to a cost saving caused by less incarceration of almost two-and-a-half million dollars ($2,497,993). This figure probably is an underestimate, because it does not take into account a reduction in the size of facilities that can further extend the savings. Also, the figure of two-and-a-half million dollars does not include the reduction in costs for the victims.

It should be noted that the additional intervention at age 14 which focused on known violent offenders, compared to the intervention focusing on at-risk youth at a young age, further reduced the percentage of homicide offenses committed but not the percentage of homicide victims. Moreover, the additional intervention with violent offenders at age 13 somewhat increased the benefits of reduced arrest for violence and the same for the weeks of incarceration (21.7% vs. 29.9%, or 142.7 years). This translates into a saving of more three million three hundred thousand dollars ($3,309,784).

Question 3: *What is the yield of an intervention at 14 based on arrest for violence without an intervention at an earlier age?* It can be argued that few communities have the resources to mount an early intervention program *and* an intervention focusing on youth arrested for violence. Instead, some communities may want to focus on an intervention that focuses on arrestees for violence only rather than trying to intervene at a young age on the basis of disruptive/delinquent behavior. How well did the intervention 2 perform without the prior Intervention 1? Figure 9.5 and Table 9.1 shows the results of the intervention following Screen 2 (arrest for violence). The age–crime curve for arrest for violence is only a little lower than that for no intervention, reflecting the fact that the reduction in arrest for violence was a mere 7.6%, which was concentrated between ages 14 and 21, thus not earlier or later. Intervention following Screen 2 only led to a 10.8% reduction in homicide offenders, a 15.4% reduction in homicide victims, and a 7.8% reduction in weeks of incarceration.

---

[4] Again, the incarceration data are based on the youngest and oldest cohorts only.

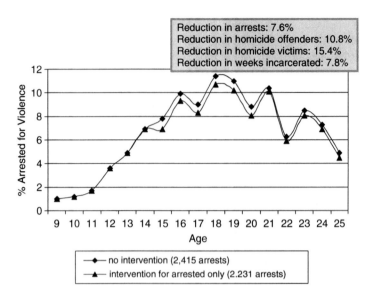

Fig. 9.5 Age–crime curve for percent arrested for violence before and after intervention on participants arrested by age 14 for violence only (youngest, middle, and oldest cohorts)

Table 9.1 Comparison of the yield of different interventions

	Target groups for interventions		
	Intervention 1: High-risk boys at a young age	Intervention 1 and 2 in sequence: High-risk boys at a young age AND boys arrested for violence at age 14	Intervention 2 alone: Boys arrested for violence at age 14
Reduction in arrest	20.0	26.8	6.9
Reduction in homicide offenders	29.7	40.5	10.8
Reduction in homicide victims	25.6	28.2	2.6
Reduction in weeks incarcerated	27.1	29.9	8.2

In summary, Screen 1 based on a risk score (child, mother, and teacher information of child problem behavior) at a young age produced substantially higher benefits in the reduction of offending, victimization, and incarceration than Screen 2 (police information of arrest for violence) by age 14. However, it should be noted that an early compared to a later intervention inherently means a higher accrual of offenses.

Question 4: *How well do the two interventions compare when serious delinquency is the outcome?* Thus far, the outcomes considered are different indicators of violence based on official records. The unanswered question is whether interventions based on Screen 1, Screen 2, or in combination reduced serious delinquency, defined

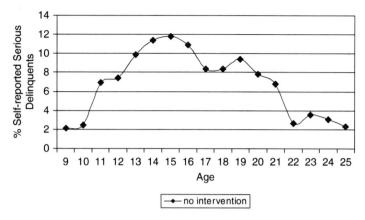

Fig. 9.6 Age–crime curve of self-reported serious delinquents without intervention (youngest and oldest samples)

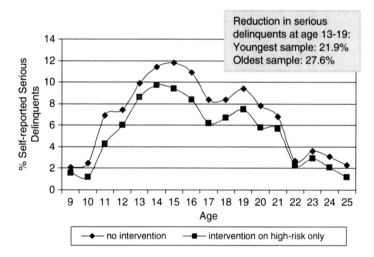

Fig. 9.7 Age–crime curve of self-reported delinquency before and after intervention on high-risk participants only (youngest and oldest cohorts)

as violence and serious theft? The indicator of serious delinquency that we will use is a best estimate of offending, based on boys' self-reports, information from parents and teachers, and records of conviction for serious delinquent acts (called the all-source measure of serious delinquency). Because this measure was not available for the middle cohort (due to the restricted follow-up of that sample), the age–crime curve for the all-source measure of serious delinquency could be computed for the youngest and oldest cohorts only. The results are summarized in Figs. 9.6–9.9. Figure 9.6 shows the age–crime curve for the prevalence of the all-source measure of serious delinquency for the youngest and oldest cohorts without the intervention. The curve increases between ages 10 and 15, peaks at age 15, and then decreases gradually to a low age at ages 22–25.

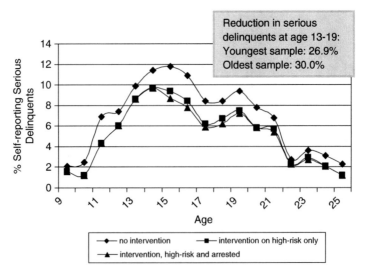

Fig. 9.8 Age–crime curve of change in self-reported serious delinquents before and after intervention on high-risk participants, followed by intervention on participants arrested by age 14 for violence (youngest and oldest samples)

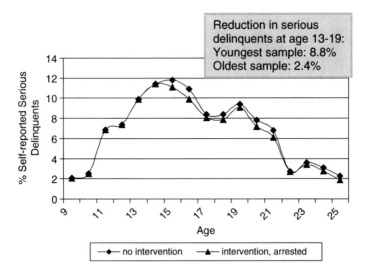

Fig. 9.9 Age–crime curve of self-reported delinquents before and after intervention on participants arrested by age 14 for violence (youngest and oldest samples)

How much is the curve lowered as a result of the first intervention at a young age? This is shown in Fig. 9.7, which demonstrates a substantial lowering of the age–crime curve as a result of the intervention, with an increasing differential after age 12 and a narrowing differential after age 15. By age 21, the differential has become very small, indicating little impact of the intervention past this age. The peak age of the age–crime curve at age 15 is lowered as a result of the intervention from a prevalence of 12% to a prevalence of below 10%, or just under one-third of the serious offenders. Lower percentages apply to the ages prior to age 15 and the ages following age 15. The reduction in serious delinquents was 21.5% for the youngest cohort, and 27.6% for the oldest cohort. Thus, the intervention has a substantial benefit of lowering the age–crime curve by reducing the prevalence of serious offenders, many of whom are outside of the purview of the justice system.

Does the added intervention based on those arrested for violence further lower the age–crime curve? The results shown in Fig. 9.8 indicate that this is not the case. At the highest differential between the interventions aimed at high-risk boys and the intervention aimed at boys arrested for violence, there is a reduction at age 15 of serious delinquents from 12% to about 10%, and the differential is even smaller subsequent to that age (the intervention differential does not apply to a younger age because it was modeled at age 14). However, the total reduction in serious delin-quents was 26.9% and 30.0% for the youngest and oldest cohorts, respectively. Thus, the yield of the second intervention over the first intervention was small.

The low impact of the second intervention is also evident from Fig. 9.9, which compares the age–crime curve for serious delinquency with no intervention against the age–crime curve for serious delinquency as a result of the second intervention. The findings demonstrate that an intervention aimed solely at boys arrested for vio-lence at age 14 does not lower the age–crime curve in a substantive manner (dif-ferential is 8.8% and 2.4% for the youngest and oldest cohorts, respectively).

Question 5: *Does an intervention at a young age (e.g., age 7 for the youngest cohort) have a higher yield in reducing the frequency of serious delinquency than an intervention at age 13 (for the oldest cohort)?* Turning back to the interventions with boys at a young age, it can be argued that the impact of interventions varies with age and that the earlier the intervention the higher its impact. On the other hand, it can also be argued that the high-risk population who eventually commits serious forms of delinquency may not have crystallized at age 7 but may emerge at a later age. In contrast, however, it can be argued that the impact of an intervention at a young age reduces more offenders, victims, and offenses down the age-line, with these numbers being inevitably smaller at a later age.

The preceding results report on the prevalence of serious offenders. It can be argued that what is more important than a reduction in the prevalence of offenders is a reduction in the offense rate or frequency. We know that the most serious delinquents often commit delinquent acts at a higher rate than the less serious delinquents. The question is to what extent an intervention reduces the frequency of serious delinquent acts in a population. Because the all-source measure of offending had been constructed as a prevalence measure, and because it does not make sense to add the frequency of convictions to the frequency of self-reported offenses, we will concentrate here on the frequency of self-reported delinquency alone.

Table 9.2 summarizes the results. First, it should be noted that the frequency of serious offenses was two-and-a-half times larger for the oldest compared to the youngest cohort between ages 13 and 19 (3,939 vs. 1,551). An early intervention at ages 7 for the youngest cohort and age 13 for the oldest cohort, produced a 21.9%

Table 9.2 Comparison between the yields of interventions at age 7 vs. 13.

| | % Reduction in frequency of serious offenses at ages | | |
	9–12	13–19	9–19
Intervention 1 at age 7 – Youngest cohort	279 – 188 = 91 (32.6%)	1,551 – 1,211 = 340 (21.9%)	1,830 – 1,302 = 528 (28.9%)
Intervention 1 at age 13 – Oldest cohort	N/A	3,939 – 2,848 = 1,091 (27.7%)	N/A

reduction in the number of serious offenses in the youngest cohort, and a 27.7% reduction in the oldest cohort, a difference of 6.2%, thus slightly larger for the oldest compared to the youngest cohort.

It can be argued that an early (age 7) compared to a later (age 13) intervention has the advantage of reducing serious offenses between ages 7 and 13. For that reason, we computed the reduction of serious offenses for the youngest cohort between ages 9 and 12 (frequency measures at an earlier age were not available due to the type of instrument used for young boys). The reduction amounted to 32.6% (see Table 9.2). Thus, one of the advantages of an early compared to a later intervention is the longer time-window that is available for the early intervention to have an impact on reducing the number of serious offenses. Table 9.2 shows that the impact of an intervention at age 7 on subsequent offending (over ages 9–12 and 13–19) for the youngest cohort reduces serious offenses by 28.9%, which is only marginally different from that observed for the oldest cohort (27.7%) in a shorter time-window (ages 13–19). Thus, the results do not clearly demonstrate that an early intervention has major advantages of reducing the frequency of serious delinquency when the timing of interventions are compared at age 7 vs. age 13. There are several caveats that need to be taken into account, which we will discuss below.

Conclusions

The first question raised was *To what extent does an intervention with a success rate of 30% that focused on high-risk boys at a young age (ages 7–13; Screen 1) reduce arrests for violence as shown in the age–crime curve, and other indicators of violent offending and incarceration?* The results of the intervention at a young age showed a substantial lowering of the age–crime curve for arrest of violence, a third of the homicide offenders and homicide victims, and a reduction in incarceration by 107 years, which amounts to a large cost saving. An important point here is that an intervention program focused on at-risk youth can have the potential to lower the age–crime curve for arrest. A study by Cook and his colleagues (2005) estimated that reducing the risk of homicide by felons to that of the general population would lead to approximately a 31% reduction in homicides. This reduction is similar to the findings of our study. We see this as a first step in the lowering of community crime levels, but only if programs can affect multiple age–crime curves of successive birth cohorts of youth.

The second question addressed: *Does an intervention at age 14 only based on arrest for violence have sufficient benefits if an intervention already has taken place at an earlier age?* The results failed to show that the two-pronged intervention focusing first on youth at ages 7–13 and then on youth arrested for violence at age 14 had a substantially higher yield than a single intervention on youth at risk for delinquency at a young age.

The third question addressed: *What is the yield of an intervention at 14 based on arrest for violence without an intervention at an earlier age?* We found that a single intervention at age 14 that focused on arrested violent offenders only did not have large yields in terms of a lowering of the age–crime curve for arrest for violence, and did not materially reduce homicide offenders, homicide victims, or the incarceration time.

The fourth question asked: *How well do the two interventions compare when serious delinquency is the outcome?* The results basically replicated the results for violence in that intervention at an early age based on the at-risk status of youth yielded a lowering of the age–crime curve for serious delinquency, and a reduction in homicide offenders and homicide victims.

The fifth inquiry addressed: *Does an intervention at a young age (e.g., age 7 for the youngest cohort) have a higher yield in reducing the frequency of offending than an intervention at age 13 (for the oldest cohort)?* It should be kept in mind that the prevalence and frequency of serious delinquency was substantially higher for the oldest than for the youngest cohort (Loeber et al., 2008). To answer this question, we limited the comparison in the reduction of offending to age period 13–19, which was the age range shared by the two cohorts. The results showed that the intervention based on the screen at age 13 reduced the frequency of offending at ages 13–19 slightly more than when the intervention was applied to a screen at age 7 (about a 6% difference in favor of the oldest cohort). However, this differential disappeared if the earlier years (ages 9–12) for the youngest cohort were taken into account as well. Thus, an intervention based on an early identification at age 7 produced a similar benefit compared with an intervention of the same strength based on an identification of at-risk boys at age 13.

Limitations

The promising results, especially for early interventions, however, should be interpreted with caution. Not all programs will have a 30% success rate, and the yields would be smaller if the success rate of programs was lower. Also, the effectiveness of programs may be lower for youth with a higher compared to a lower propensity for delinquency and violence.

There are several other caveats. First, the assumption is that screens at age 7 and age 13 are equivalent in their power to identify high-risk boys. There is some reason to doubt this, but it would require other types of analyses to sort this out completely.

Second, the percentage reduction in the prevalence of offending is probably not as good a measure as a reduction in the frequency of offending, because a larger compared to a smaller reduction in frequency (as in the case of the oldest cohort) obviously benefits communities more as victimization rates go down. The percentage reduction in the frequency of serious delinquency amounted to very different absolute numbers in the youngest vs. the oldest cohort, with the reduction in the total number of serious delinquent acts being the highest in the oldest cohort which was the most delinquent of the two cohorts. In addition, as mentioned before, the projected reduction in offending is a function of the efficacy of intervention, rising when the efficacy increases and decreasing when the efficacy becomes less. Lastly, we compared ages 7 vs. 13 in terms of intervention applied to at-risk categories of boys. It remains to be seen whether interventions below age 7, or between ages 7 and 13 would have different yields than the interventions modeled here.

There are several other limitations to the two simulation studies. Data on violence and homicide are based only on the PYS. This study is remarkable for its longitudinal nature, its population-based sampling, and the great efforts taken to limit attrition among study participants, which has enabled investigators to track youths from childhood until 25 years of age (Stouthamer-Loeber, Loeber, & Thomas, 1992). Nonetheless, these individuals represent urban males from one geographic location and may not be representative of other males, including rural populations facing very different environmental and cultural contexts. Nonetheless, most homicides are committed by urban male youths not unlike the Pittsburgh cohorts.

We have regretfully excluded females from this study, given the limited data on effective intervention programs for violence involving females and the fact that the linkages between female childhood physical aggression and adolescent offending are much less established (Broidy et al., 2003; Loeber et al., 1998).

Estimations of program effectiveness were based on reductions in arrest rates for criminal and violent acts combined with data linking arrests to the development of later violent crimes and homicide. While it would be preferable to study homicide rates as an outcome of an intervention study, this is unlikely to be practical given the long follow-up time and sample size required.

It is clear that the precursors to male violent behaviors very often begin in childhood, that there are clearly identifiable risk factors (Chaps. 4 and 5, this volume; Hawkins, Laub, & Lauritsen, 1998; Lipsey & Derzon, 1998; Loeber et al., 2005a), and that effective programs exist for preventing and treating violence (Loeber & Farrington, 2001). The present analyses suggest that implementation of these programs could potentially avert significant costs in human lives, safety and security, and economic losses that result from violent crime. Does the political and fiscal will exist to consider national implementation of tested and effective youth-focused violence prevention programs as a key element of rational violence prevention policy in the USA?

Chapter 10
Conclusions and Implications

Rolf Loeber and David P. Farrington

This volume is unique in that it focuses on the childhood and adolescence of several high-risk populations, including homicide offenders, violent offenders in general, homicide victims, and shooting victims. Although there is a growing number of books on homicide (e.g., Brookman, 2005; Heide, 2003; Holinger, Offer, Barter, & Bell, 1994; Kelly & Totten, 2002; Roth, 2009), to our knowledge this is the first book ever published based on a major longitudinal prospective study of a general population sample of young boys first studied in their childhood and adolescent years before any of them became a killer or a victim of homicide. This is in contrast with earlier studies which usually were based on small, special populations of homicide offenders with very restricted case–control or no control comparisons and reliance on retrospective rather than the more reliable and comprehensive prospective information (see the studies cited in Chap. 1). Another unique aspect of this volume is the fact that we can compare the criminal history and exposure to risk factors of homicide offenders with violent, nonhomicidal offenders, homicide victims, and shooting victims. Thus, the long-term prospective follow-up of young boys chronicled in this volume also fills a major gap in the scientific literature by focusing on a wide range of prospective risk factors related to homicide and shooting victims, on which very little has been published.

Unlike many other prior studies that relied on retrospective reports, this volume is based on prospective information collected at least yearly over a decade or more about the background and behavioral development of convicted homicide offenders and homicide victims. In addition, the book provides detailed information about a third and a fourth group, namely those who were arrested for homicide but not convicted, and those who were shot but who did not die. The present book was written to stimulate the debate on what policy makers on the national, state, and city government levels should do to reduce the homicide rate in the USA, since that is much higher than in most other developed nations.

Each of the preceding chapters addressed key questions and we will now return to these questions, summarize our findings, and review their implications for interventions and policy. At the end of this chapter will also address other key issues raised in the Introduction, such as the relevance of the findings for theories about homicide offending and victimization, whether screening for homicide offenders and victims is feasible, and whether incarceration for homicide offenders is better than prevention. Finally, we will address which future policies are needed to reduce homicides involving young people. Before doing so, we will briefly state the limitations of this volume.

Limitations

There are several limitations that apply to this volume. It mostly concerns "street" violence and homicide and does not focus on intimate partner homicide, largely because very few of the young men in the PYS murdered their partners. Although biological factors, such as peripheral neurological functioning, head trauma, brain development, and brain functioning, have been hypothesized to be important in violence and homicide (e.g., Heide, 2004; Loeber, Pardini, Stouthamer-Loeber, & Raine, 2007; Raine, 1993), we could not pursue these topics in this volume. Such factors are currently being investigated in the youngest and oldest cohorts of the PYS, but the data are not yet available. The same applies to genetic data, which also are currently being collected.

Second, the investigation of homicide offending is hampered by the fact that the study of immediate circumstances and decision processes of homicide offenders are beyond the scope of this study, and by necessity need to be reconstructed from police accounts and retrospective information from perpetrators (see, e.g., Wikström & Treiber, 2009). The investigation of homicide victimization is even more limited in that information about the immediate situation is often based on police accounts only.

Weighing against these study limitations, however, are the many strengths of the current study. First is the fact that many waves of systematically collected data were available on the violent offenders, homicide offenders, homicide victims, and shooting victims. These data came from multiple informants, including the parents, teachers, the young males themselves, the school test data, police, and courts. A particular advantage of the data are the repeated measurements of a large array of risk factors (the first assessment took place in 1987 when the participants were aged 7–13, and most of them were regularly followed up until their twenties), and a larger number of homicide offenders (see below) than was available in an earlier paper (Loeber et al., 2005a). We will start by reviewing the violent offenders because the majority of the homicide offenders emerged over time from the violent offenders.

Homicide Offenders

How common are homicide crimes in Pittsburgh, and how does this compare regionally and nationally? As shown in Chap. 3, by May 2009, out of the 1,517 boys in the Pittsburgh Youth Study (PYS; described in Chap. 2), 37 had been convicted in court for committing a homicide. Given that the PYS consisted of an enriched sample (with oversampling of high-risk boys), the weighted corrected, life-time rate was 2.0 boys per 100 (or prorated 1,984 per 100,000 young males). As shown in Chap. 3, the rate of homicide offenders in the PYS is twice as high as that for African Americans in the age 18–24 age range in the USA, which is eight times higher than for Caucasian males.

How representative are homicide offenders in the PYS compared to homicide offenders in Allegheny County (where Pittsburgh is located), Pennsylvania, and the USA? Even though this book chronicles the lives of homicide offenders and homicide victims in Pittsburgh, we demonstrated in Chap. 3 (and later in Chap. 7) that for the great majority of the homicide offenders in that city, the circumstances under which homicide is committed (arguments, guns, gangs, African American males, disadvantaged neighborhoods) and the characteristics of their homicide victims (Chap. 3) are very similar to those in other major cities. Most of the killings were accomplished by means of a firearm and took place in the most disadvantaged neighborhoods (see also Nieuwbeerta, McCall, Elffers, & Wittebrood, 2008).

Homicides by young males in the PYS were a microcosm of homicides on the county, city, and national level. Other key similarities are a high overrepresentation of African American young males among both offenders and victims. Most of them, prior to the homicide, were known to the police and the court and tended to have a criminal record. Virtually all homicide offenders only committed a single homicide, and multiple killings were rare (see also Block & Block, 2008). Intra-racial killing was the norm. These and other comparisons in Chap. 3 support the notion that homicide offenders and their homicides in the PYS are largely representative of homicide offenders and their homicides at the broader local and national levels. Thus, we are confident that conclusions drawn from the present study are relevant to the much wider phenomena of homicide in many of the major cities in the USA.

What is the most common type of homicide offender in this study? Results presented in Chaps. 3 and 7 show that the great majority of the homicides committed by PYS young males, like the homicides in other major inner city, metropolitan areas, can be characterized as "street" homicides involving acquaintances and strangers rather than homicides of relatives committed by individuals "engaging in dangerous, violent behavior," resulting in death (Kelly & Totten, 2002, p. 146). Street homicide committed in the course of other criminal activity is known as "felony homicide" (Benedek & Cornell, 1989, p. 63). Another common element is that the offender and the victim attempt to gain an advantage over each other, resulting in the homicide (Decker, 1996).

What were the circumstances surrounding the homicide crimes, motives of offenders, and weapons used? Chapters 3 and 7 present findings on this. The study of circumstances surrounding the homicides was hampered by the availability of second-hand information only, although somewhat firmed up by later detailed interviews with the homicide offenders after the homicide events (Chap. 7). The most common reasons given were a robbery gone badly, self-defense in the course of being robbed, and an argument that had got out of hand. Less common reasons were drug deals, gang victimization and vehicle accidents. The majority of the homicides were committed by means of a gun, and rarely by means of a knife or an object of convenience. Two-thirds of the homicides were committed with co-offenders being present. Two-thirds of the homicide offenders reported having used drugs before the offense, with marijuana being the most common drug. In less than half of the instances, homicide offenders had consumed alcohol prior to the offense. It should be noted that research indicates that, although marijuana use is correlated with violence, alcohol is much more important as an antecedent to violence (White, Loeber, Stouthamer-Loeber, & Farrington, 1999).

The detailed interviews showed that three quarters of the homicide offenders knew their victim. Feelings of fear rather than aggression were predominant prior to the homicide: one-third reported no feelings, another third reported feeling fear, and one-fifth felt angry. Subsequently, feelings of fear were the predominant emotion after the homicide. Although we do not know the object of fear, it is likely that homicide offenders fear detection and retribution.

Explanatory, Behavioral and Criminal Risk Factors. Both prior criminal offenses and early behavior problems can be thought as manifestations of rule breaking and antisocial behavior in general. For that reason, we distinguished these behaviors from explanatory factors thought to be more independent from homicide offending and violence in general. The key question here was: *Which explanatory, behavioral, and criminal risk factors predict homicide offenders out of a community sample up to 22 years later?*

Explanatory Predictors. In Chap. 4 we found that 9 out of 21 explanatory factors predicted convicted homicide offenders. The strongest factors in a regression analysis were broken home, the family on welfare, and a young mother. These structural factors, rather than imperfect childrearing practices or association with delinquent peers, were the best predictors of homicide offenders.

Behavioral Predictors. To what extent did homicide offenders engage in antisocial and delinquent behavior earlier in life? We found that 95% of the convicted homicide offenders were known to have been violent earlier in life (see Chap. 5). In addition, the interviews with homicide offenders reported in Chap. 7 documented situational factors proximal to the homicide. Compared to controls, almost all (89%) of the homicide offenders had engaged in drug dealing (4% for controls), three quarters (74%) had engaged in recent serious violence, and fewer (15%) had engaged in serious theft.

The only summary psychiatric diagnosis we could investigate was Disruptive Behavior Disorder, which means that an individual qualified for a DSM-IIIR diagnosis of one or more of the following disorders: Attention Deficit Hyperactivity Disorder, Conduct Disorder or Oppositional Defiant Disorder. Results reported in Chap. 4 show that Disruptive Behavior Disorder survived in a logistic regression of the behavioral predictors of convicted homicide offenders and, importantly, also featured as one of the predictors in the final, integrated prediction score for homicide offenders. Thus, significantly more of the homicide offenders compared to the controls qualified for a diagnosis of Disruptive Behavior Disorder when young. However, because delinquency overlaps with the criteria for Conduct Disorder (one of the three disorders comprising Disruptive Behavior Disorders), this indicates that many future homicide offenders showed earlier behavior problems (see also Hagelstam & Häkkänen, 2006). We cannot conclude that Disruptive Behavior Disorder had any causal effect on later homicide offending. Finally, we were not able to investigate psychosis among the homicide offenders; however, other studies show that psychosis is very rare among adolescent homicide offenders (e.g., Benedek & Cornell, 1989).

Several other behavioral markers emerged from the prediction analyses. The results of regression analyses reported in Chap. 4 show that suspension from school, a positive attitude to delinquency, a high screening risk score (indicative of general acting-out behaviors at a young age), and a diagnosis of Disruptive Behavior Disorder were the best independent predictors of convicted homicide offenders.

We infer that in the majority of cases homicide offending is the culmination of individuals' progress on three pathways from childhood to adolescence and early adulthood (Loeber et al., 1993; Loeber, Lacourse, & Homish, 2005): (a) The Authority Conflict Pathway leading to conflict with authority figures (parents and teachers) to avoidance of control by these adults; (b) the Overt Pathway of escalating violence starting with lesser forms of problem aggression; and (c) the Covert Pathway consisting of an escalation from less serious covert acts (such as frequent lying and shoplifting) to serious forms of property crime. We argue that for the majority of the homicide offenders in the PYS, their progress on the three pathways prepared them early in life to become versatile rather than specialized offenders. This conclusion is also strengthened by the fact that both violent offenses and property offenses predicted convicted homicide offenders (discussed below).

Criminal Predictors. We studied a wide range of offense types measured by means of self-reports, arrests, and convictions. In univariate analyses reported in Chap. 4 and summarized in Table 10.2, we found that 57 types of offending, covering violence, property crime, drug crime, and other categories, predicted homicide offenders. The self-reported offenses prior to age 15 which in logistic regression analyses best predicted homicide offending were vehicle theft and weapon carrying, followed by violence, minor fraud (avoid paying), robbery, a total theft index, drug selling, vandalism, and theft from a car. Thus a range of prior violent, but also property, offenses predicted convicted homicide offenders. Not all of these offenses were known to justice officials. For that reason, we also examined offenses based on official records compared to self-report. The results show that convictions or arrests for various forms of violence were a better predictor of homicide offending than were self-reports of violence. In addition, convictions for receiving stolen goods were a better predictor than were self-reports of the same act. This supports the notion, which we will develop later while discussing explanatory theories, that engagement in the illicit or underground economy is a precursor to some young males eventually becoming a homicide offender or a homicide victim.

To what extent can convicted homicide offenders be predicted based on a combination of explanatory, behavioral, and criminal risk factors? The integrated analyses were based on factors that were independent and statistically significant in each of the three preceding regression analyses (explanatory, behavioral, and criminal).

The results reported in Chap. 4 showed that factors from three domains (individual, family, and neighborhood) independently contributed to the prediction of homicide offenders. These factors included prior delinquent acts, including conviction for other/conspiracy (a general category of offenses), simple assault, and weapon carrying; living in a bad neighborhood, and having a young mother. Thus, no single factor could best explain or predict homicide offenders.

Instead, we addressed the question: *Is there a dose–response relationship between the number of risk factors and the probability of becoming a homicide offender?* The integrated homicide risk score reported in Chap. 4 for the prediction of convicted homicide offenders from the whole population showed a dose–response relationship between the number of risk factors and the probability of becoming a offenders: the higher the number of risk factors, the higher the probability of a homicide offender. None of the boys who scored zero on the risk factors became a homicide offender compared to 19% who had 5–7 risk factors. AUC analyses show good predictability (AUC=.870) at a level that was higher than for explanatory, behavioral, and criminal risk factors alone. Not surprisingly the false-positive error rate was high (87%), indicating overprediction, while the false-negative error rate (38%) was moderately high, indicating that almost four out of ten homicide offenders were not indentified on the basis of the prediction score.

Estimating True Prediction. Because the constituent variables in the prediction analyses were chosen in the light of knowledge about which were the best predictors of homicide offenders, the predictive efficiency may have been overestimated in the prior analyses. For that reason, we compared in Chap. 4 the prediction of the screening risk score (which was not based on prior knowledge) with that of the behavioral risk score. The results showed that an unbiased AUC based on the behavioral risk score might of the order of .72 to .75 and that an unbiased OR might be of the order of 5.

Are homicide offenders predominantly psychopaths? The negative findings in the prediction of homicide offenders (Chap. 4) are equally important as the positive findings. For example, we did not find in the regression analyses in Chap. 4 that factors typically associated with psychopathy were predictive of homicide offenders. These factors were lack of guilt, cruelty to people and callous-unemotional behavior.[1] However, interviews with homicide offenders (Chap. 7) using the Psychopathy Checklist – Screening Version (PCL-SV) showed that three quarters of them scored high on all PCL-SV factors. These results were largely driven by higher scores on Factors 3 (impulsiveness and irresponsible lifestyle) and 4 (juvenile delinquency and criminal versatility) and not on the crucial personality Factors 1 (arrogance and deceitfulness) and 2 (lack of empathy and guilt). Thus, there was little evidence suggesting that the homicide offenders were predominantly psychopaths. However, we cannot state that this question is fully resolved. Chapter 7 had missing data which may have affected the results. Also, prediction analyses of violent offenders reported in Chap. 5 indicate that among the best predictors were callous-unemotional behavior and lack of guilt.

---

[1] However, in univariate analyses (summarized in Table 10.1) we found that lack of guilt was a predictor of convicted homicide offenders.

Do predictors recorded in childhood continue to predict convicted homicide offenders even when predictors recorded in adolescence are taken into account? To address this question, we examined whether predictors measured in childhood (i.e., age 7 in the youngest cohort; age 10 in the middle cohort; and age 13 in the oldest cohort) predicted homicide offenders when controlling for later predictors measured in adolescence. The logistic regression analysis showed that three explanatory factors measured in childhood (a bad neighborhood, a young mother, and an unemployed mother) continued to predict homicide offenders even when earlier behavioral factors and later factors measured in adolescence were taken into account. We interpret this to show that the processes leading to homicide offending are partly present in childhood but that factors which emerge in adolescence, such as a positive attitude to substance use and problem behavior that leads to school suspension, further increase the probability of young males committing homicide later. The results argue against the notion that all etiological factors pertaining to homicide are already in place during childhood.

Is the prediction of homicide offenders more efficient when based on those who were violent earlier in life compared to a prediction based on the general population of youth? A comparison of the results in Chaps. 4 and 5 showed that this was not the case. We had expected that the step-wise prediction (first predicting violence and then predicting homicide offenders out of the violent offenders) would not only increase the base-rate of homicide offenders but also improve the predictive efficacy, and lower false-positive errors and lower false-negative errors. The results presented in Chap. 5 indicate that the percentage of convicted homicide offenders among high-risk violent boys was very similar to the percentage of convicted homicide offenders among boys in the total sample with high behavioral risk scores (20 and 17%, respectively). Also, the predictive efficacy (as expressed by AUC) was very similar in both methods. In addition, the proportion of false-negative errors resulting from the step-wise prediction was only slightly better than that based on whole population prediction (30% vs. 38%), while the false-positive errors were in the same range (89% vs. 87%). We speculate that the predictive accuracy reported in Chaps. 4 and 5 may be close to the maximum possible, given the unpredictability of homicide convictions. On the more positive side, screening for violence appears more feasible (see, e.g., Loeber et al., 2005a), which we will discuss below.

Homicide Arrestees

Not all individuals arrested for homicide are guilty. At the same time, it is possible that some arrestees are actually homicide offenders but because of lack of evidence, escape being convicted. In Chap. 4 we reported that 33 boys were arrested for homicide but not (yet) convicted. However, if most arrestees were genuinely not guilty of homicide, they would share few if any risk factors. To address this issue, we asked: *To what extent were the homicide arrestees exposed to the same childhood risk factors as the convicted homicide offenders?* For that reason, we compared homicide arrestees with homicide offenders on their exposure to risk factors. We expected that if the two categories of offenders were similar, they would share many risk factors. Out of 40 explanatory and behavioral risk factors in childhood, 16 predicted homicide arrestees. However, we found little overlap between the predictors of homicide arrestees and homicide offenders. Also, the best predictors of homicide arrestees predicted less well than the best predictors of homicide offenders. The results indicate that homicide arrestees and homicide offenders were largely different groups.

Violent Offenders

Before turning to the homicide victims, we briefly discuss issues surrounding violent offenders. As mentioned, 95% of the homicide offenders had been violent earlier in life. Thus, it is probable that prior violence is a stepping-stone to homicide offending, with the understanding that only a minority of the violent offenders makes the transition to become a homicide offender. Because this volume focuses on homicide offenders and homicide victims, the following summary of findings will be relatively brief. For a more extensive treatment of violent offenders in the PYS, the reader is referred to Loeber et al. (2005a) and Loeber, Farrington, Stouthamer-Loeber, and White (2008).

Prevalence. As we reviewed in Chap. 5, violence was endemic in Pittsburgh: out of all boys half were violent according to official records or self-reports. Analyses reported by Loeber et al. (2008) indicate that the persistence of violence is higher than the persistence of property offenses.

Predictors of Violence. Research indicates that a range of early behavior problems predict violence (Farrington, 1998; Loeber et al., 1993). For example, Huebner, Varano, and Bynum (2007) studied future offending in a sample of 322 young men aged 17–24 years released from prison, and showed that race, gang membership, drug dependence, and institutional behavior were critical predictors but not the type of weapon used, possibly because gun use was very common.

In Chap. 5 we presented the best "predictors" of violence. The caveat here is, however, that in contrast to the Loeber et al. (2005a) paper, the temporal priority of predictors of violence could not be fully adhered to. We studied a wider range of risk factors because we included risk factors in adolescence as well. Thus, the meaning of "predictors" in the case of violent offenders is less strict here than for predictors of homicide offenders and homicide victims in the remainder of this volume.

The results show that 58 out of 59 risk factors, representing all measurement domains, significantly predicted violent offenders. For example, 23% of the violent young men had been exposed to recorded child abuse, compared to 9% of the controls. It should be noted that child abuse (at least evident from the official records), although a predictor of violence, was experienced by only a quarter of the violent offenders. The strongest explanatory factors were callous-unemotional behavior, lack of guilt, an index of hyperactivity–impulsivity–attention problems, and broken home. The following behavioral factors were strongest: prior serious delinquency, selling hard drugs or marijuana, gun carrying, nonphysical aggression, and gang fighting. These predictors largely replicate those found for violence in other longitudinal studies (Farrington, 1998; Hawkins, Laub, & Lauritsen, 1998; Lipsey & Derzon, 1998).

Violence Risk Score. Based on the regression results, we constructed a violence risk score based on the best predictors of violence. Results presented in Chap. 5 confirm that there is a dose–response relationship: the higher the number of risk factors, the higher the probability of becoming a violent offender. The percentage violent offenders increased from 8% of those with no risk factors to 100% of those with ten or more risk factors. The AUC of .832 was substantial, indicating strong predictive efficacy.

Homicide Victims

The study of the behavioral background of homicide offenders traditionally has been distinct from the study of the behavioral background of homicide victims, largely because of problems in reconstructing the lives of victims before being killed. The present volume, because of the unique availability of prospective longitudinal data on homicide offenders and homicide victims, sheds light on the many antecedent factors in the lives of each. Similar proportions of this community sample of young males became convicted homicide offenders (2.4%) and homicide victims (about 2.6%). There is another major advantage of this volume in that we consider the similarities of the lives of homicide offenders and homicide victims as crucial in advancing homicide studies. Thus, it is the shared risks in their earlier life and the shared criminal activities (Lauritsen, Sampson, & Laub, 1991) that can provide unique insights into process that brings homicide offenders and their victims together for the fatal act. In this section, we will address several pertinent questions that highlight this joint phenomenon of offending and victimization.

To what extent did homicide victims engage in antisocial behaviors? As mentioned when discussing street crime, the majority of victims had engaged in delinquent behavior prior to their death. Compared to controls, the homicide victims were more likely to have carried a gun, to have used a weapon to attack someone, engaged in gang fights or committed a robbery. They also had been more involved in gang fights and were more likely to have sold marijuana or hard drugs.

In summary, the results presented in Chap. 6 shows that the majority of homicide victims had a history of law breaking, especially engagement in illicit activities such as receiving stolen property, stealing cars, or stealing from a car (in addition, aggravated assault was one of the predictors of homicide victimization). Thus, the activities of the homicide offenders and the homicide victims often centered around frequent delinquent acts, engaging in the black economy by dealing in stolen goods and, for the homicide offenders, drug dealing. It is likely that the administration of personal justice to deal with conflicts arising from these transactions "in the street" and gang membership for a proportion of the offenders further fuels victimization and retaliation. This is aided by the fact that the most delinquents living in disadvantaged neighborhoods when themselves victimized tend to underreport their victimization to the police (Berg, Slocum, & Loeber, 2011). Instead, the victimization of innocent bystanders is most well-known to the police and receives the most media attention.

Which explanatory, behavioral, and criminal risk factors predict homicide victims out of a community sample up to 22 years later? Among the strongest explanatory factors were lack of guilt, low achievement on the California Achievement Test, broken home, and large family size. The strongest behavioral predictors of homicide victims were serious delinquency, a bad relationship with a parent, and physical aggression. Turning to criminal predictors, the strongest predictors were vehicle theft, aggravated assault, theft from a car, and receiving stolen property (all self-reported), drug offenses, vehicle theft, and receiving property (all according to criminal convictions), receiving stolen property, vehicle theft, and drug offenses (all according to arrest data). Thus, predominantly property offenses predicted homicide victims, particularly receiving stolen goods, vehicle theft, and theft from a vehicle. Thus, more of the homicide victims, compared to the controls, appear to have participated in the black economy including the acquisition and sale of stolen goods.

Is there a dose–response relationship between the number of risk factors and the probability of becoming a homicide victim? In Chaps. 4 and 5 we computed, using information on the best predictors in the three areas (explanatory, behavioral, and criminal) evident from logistic regression analyses, an integrated risk score to predict homicide offenders. In Chap. 6 we did the same but with homicide victims as the outcome. Less than 1% of those boys with zero or one risk factor became a homicide victim, compared to 17% with 4–6 risk factors. The results show that the higher the number of risk factors the higher the probability of becoming a homicide victim. However, predictive efficiency at three or more risk factors was modest (see below).

In Chap. 6 we also emphasized that predictive accuracy for homicide victims is overestimated because the constituent variables were chosen in the light of knowledge about which are the best predictors. For that reason, we chose the number of arrests up to age 14 as a predictor of homicide victims. The AUC for the number of arrests was .706 compared with .806 for the criminal risk score. Thus, it is reasonable to suggest that an unbiased AUC based on a criminal risk score might be of the order of .75, and that an unbiased OR might be about 6.

Shooting Victims

In Chap. 6 we mentioned, that out of the 1,517 young males in the study, 128 (8.4%) were shot before age 30, of whom 37 (29%) died. Of the remainder, 78 shooting victims were not arrested or convicted for homicide offending. Many of the questions pertaining to homicide victims also pertain to shooting victims.

To what extent did shooting victims engage in antisocial behaviors? Compared to controls, the shooting victims were significantly more likely to have been antisocial, including selling hard drugs, gang membership, carrying a gun, and selling marijuana.

Which explanatory, behavioral, and criminal risk factors predict shooting victims up to 22 years later? The results reported in Chap. 6 show that the most important predictors were: broken home, self-reported drug selling, low school motivation, truancy, and peer delinquency. The AUC was .733 showing moderately good predictability. The formulation of a risk score on the basis of these factors showed again a dose-relationship between the number of risk factors and the probability of young males becoming a shooting victim. Only 3% of boys with none of the risk factors became homicide victims, compared with 15% of the boys with four to five of these risk factors.

Comparing Homicide Offenders, Violent Offenders, Homicide Victims, and Shooting Victims

The four outcomes central to this volume, convicted homicide offenders, violent offenders, homicide victims, and shooting victims, are distinct groups in our analyses. In practice, membership of one rather than another group may partly depend on the type of weapon individuals carried, their willingness to use that weapon against an opponent, their marksmanship, and the ability of individuals to defend themselves against violence. Also, the probability of dying when shot depends on the type of bullet, the area of the wound(s), the loss of blood, and the speed and effectiveness of emergency help. Many young males who are shot nevertheless survive.

In Chap. 1, we mentioned that some criminologists have proposed that homicide victims and homicide offenders are "chips off the same block" and share many of the same offense characteristics and earlier risk factors. However, homicide offenders are thought to be more antisocial prior to the homicide than homicide victims.

To investigate shared predictors among offenders and victims, we summarized the main univariate findings from Chaps. 4–6 in two tables.[2] Table 10.1 shows the explanatory and behavioral predictors of violent offenders, convicted homicide offenders, homicide victims, and shooting victims. Univariate predictors are the focus here because we are particularly interested to know to what extent possible causal processes, represented by the univariate results, differ among the various categories of offenders and victims. Note that for each category of offender or victim, the comparison group may have differed slightly for each category. The statistical power of the comparisons was nearly identical for homicide offenders ($N = 37$) and homicide victims ($N = 39$), but slightly higher for shooting victims ($N = 78$), and highest for violent offenders ($N = 652$).

---

[2] This table contains some new information not presented elsewhere in this volume. Details about the new analyses can be obtained from the authors.

Table 10.1 Summary of the explanatory and behavioral risk factors predicting violent offenders, homicide offenders, homicide victims, and shooting victims (univariate results)

	Violent offenders (*N*=652)	Homicide offenders (*N*=37)	Homicide victims (*N*=39)	Shooting victims (*N*=78)
Explanatory factors				
Birth				
Prenatal problems	X	–	–	–
Mother cigarette use	X	–	–	–
Mother alcohol use	X	–	–	–
Child – Callous				
Lack of guilt	X	X	X	X
Callous-unemotional	X	–	X	X
Child – School				
HIA	X	X	X	X
Old for the grade	X	X	X	–
Low achievement (CAT)	X	–	X	X
Low achievement (PT)	X	–	X	X
Child – Mood				
Depressed mood	X	–	–	X
Shy/withdrawn	X	–	–	–
Boy not involved	X	–	–	–
Family – Functioning				
Young mother	X	X	–	X
Broken family	X	X	X	X
Father behavior problems	X	X	X	X
Parent substance use	X	–	–	X
Parent stress	X	–	–	–
Police contact relatives	X	–	–	–
Family – Childrearing				
Poor supervision	X	–	–	–
Physical punishment	X	–	–	–
Poor communication	X	–	–	–
Child abuse	X	X	X	–
Family – Socioeconomic				
Low socioeconomic status	X	X	–	X
Family on welfare	X	X	X	X
Large family size	X	–	X	–
Small house	X	–	–	–
Unemployed mother	X	X	–	X
Neighborhood				
Bad neighborhood (C)	X	X	X	X
Bad neighborhood (P)	X	–	X	X
Behavioral factors				
Child behavior				
Serious delinquency	X	X	X	X
Covert behavior	X	X	X	X
Physical aggression	X	–	X	X

(continued)

Table 10.1 (continued)

	Violent offenders (N=652)	Homicide offenders (N=37)	Homicide victims (N=39)	Shooting victims (N=78)
Nonphysical aggression	X	–	X	–
Cruel to people	X	X	X	X
Cruel to animals	X	–	–	–
Runs away	X	–	–	–
Disruptive behavior disorder	X	X	X	–
High-risk score	X	X	X	X
Child attitude				
Positive attitude to delinquency	X	X	–	–
Positive attitude to substance use	–	X	–	–
Unlikely to be caught	X	–	–	–
Parent				
Bad relationship with parent	X	–	X	–
Counter control	X	–	–	–
Peer				
Peer delinquency	X	X	X	X
Peer substance use	X	X	–	–
Bad friends	X	X	X	–
Bad relationship with peers	X	–	X	X
School				
Suspended	X	X	X	X
Truant	X	X	X	X
Negative attitude to school	X	–	–	–
Low school motivation	X	–	X	X
Offending				
Weapon carrying	X	X	–	–
Gun carrying	X	X	X	X
Weapon use	X	X	X	–
Gang membership	X	X	–	X
Gang fight	X	X	X	–
Sold marijuana	X	X	X	X
Sold hard drugs	X	X	X	X
Persistent drug use	X	X	–	–

Notes: X=significant univariate effect or OR at least 2; – nonsignificant. This table contains some new information not presented elsewhere in this volume. Details about the new analyses can be obtained from the authors

Table 10.2 Summary of significant criminal predictors of homicide offenders, homicide victims and shooting victims (univariate results)

	Violent offenders (N=652)	Homicide offenders (N=37)	Homicide victims (N=39)	Shooting victims (N=78)
Self-reported delinquency				
Violence				
Robbery	a	X	–	–
Aggravated assault	a	X	X	–
Gang fight	X	X	X	X
Violence (3)	X	X	X	X
Weapon carrying	X	X	–	X
Property				
Burglary	X	X	–	X
Vehicle theft	X	X	X	X
Theft from person	X	–	–	–
Theft from car	X	X	X	–
Theft (4)	X	X	X	X
Shoplifting	X	X	–	X
Other theft	X	–	–	X
Receiving	X	–	X	X
Arson	X	–	X	–
Vandalism	X	X	X	–
Drug				
Drug selling	X	X	X	X
Hard drug use	X	X	–	–
Marijuana use	X	X	X	X
Drug (3)	X	X	–	X
Other deviance				
Minor fraud	X	X	X	X
Drunk in public	X	–	X	X
Alcohol use	X	–	–	–
Tobacco use	X	X	–	–
Convictions				
Violence				
Robbery	a	X	–	–
Aggravated assault	a	X	–	X
Simple assault	X	X	–	–
Violence (3)	X	X	–	X
Threats	X	X	X	–
Weapons	X	X	–	–
Sex	X	X	–	–
Property				
Burglary	X	X	–	–
Vehicle theft	X	X	X	–
Larceny	X	X	X	X
Theft (3)	X	X	X	–
Receiving	X	X	X	–
Vandalism	X	X	–	–

(continued)

Table 10.2 (continued)

	Violent offenders (N=652)	Homicide offenders (N=37)	Homicide victims (N=39)	Shooting victims (N=78)
Other				
Drug	X	X	X	–
Mischief/disorder	X	X	X	X
Other/conspiracy	X	X	X	–
Any conviction	X	X	X	X
Arrest				
Violence				
Robbery	a	X	X	–
Aggravated assault	a	X	X	X
Simple assault	X	X	X	–
Violence (3)	X	X	X	–
Threats	X	X	–	–
Weapons	X	X	–	–
Sex	X	X	–	–
Property				
Burglary	X	X	–	–
Vehicle theft	X	X	X	X
Larceny	X	X	X	–
Theft (3)	X	X	X	–
Receiving	X	X	X	–
Vandalism	X	X	X	–
Other				
Drug	X	–	X	–
Mischief/disorder	X	X	X	X
Other/conspiracy	X	X	X	–
Any arrest	X	X	X	X

Notes: X=significant univariate effect or OR at least 2; – nonsignificant; [a]Logically related. This table contains some new information not presented elsewhere in this volume. Details about the new analyses can be obtained from the authors. The gang fight and weapon carrying variables in this table were cumulative measures up to age 14. The gang fight and weapon carrying variables in Table 10.1 were measured at wave E (see Table 2.3). Violence (3) is any of the three prior violence offenses. Theft (4) is any of the four prior property offenses. Drug (3) is any of the three prior drug offenses

Not surprisingly, the largest number of significant predictors was found for violent offenders, all factors except one were significant predictors. Most of the categories of predictors (child behaviors, family functioning, family childrearing, and family socioeconomic) applied to all four categories of individuals. However, whereas birth factors and childrearing practices predicted violence, these factors did not predict homicide offenders, homicide victims, or shooting victims (with one exception: child abuse).

Since virtually all predictors of violence were significant (58 out 59) it was inevitably true that virtually all significant predictors of homicide offenders (30 out of 31), homicide victims (32 out of 32), and shooting victims (29 out of 29) were subsets of the significant predictors of violence. This implies that causal processes, reflected in the significant univariate predictors, were partly shared between violent offenders and the three other outcome groups: homicide offenders, homicide victims, and shooting victims.

These findings, however, do not mean that causal processes explaining homicide offenders are the same as those explaining homicide victims or shooting victims. To what extent are there shared predictors among homicide offenders, homicide victims, and shooting victims? Of the 31 significant predictors of homicide offenders, 22 (71%) were also significant predictors of homicide victims. Conversely, of 28 nonsignificant predictors of homicide offenders, 18 (64%) were nonsignificant predictors of homicide victims. The predictors of homicide offenders and victims were significantly related (OR = 4.4, CI = 1.5–13.2). Similarly, of 31 significant predictors of homicide offenders, 20 (65%) were also significant predictors of shooting victims and, of 28 nonsignificant predictors of shooting victims of homicide offenders, 19 (68%) were nonsignificant predictors of shooting victims. The predictors of homicide offenders and shooting victims were also significantly related (OR = 3.8, CI = 1.3–11.3).

Not surprisingly, the significant predictors of homicide victims and shooting victims were the most strongly related. Of 32 significant predictors of homicide victims, 23 (72%) were also significant predictors of shooting victims. Of 27 nonsignificant predictors of homicide victims, 21 (78%) were also nonsignificant predictors of shooting victims. The OR was 8.9 (CI = 2.7–29.4). Thus, homicide offenders, homicide victims, and shooting victims share about two-thirds of the explanatory and behavioral predictors. Homicide victims and shooting victims share slightly more than two-thirds of the predictors, but this proportion is lower for the comparisons between homicide offenders and homicide victims and between homicide victims and shooting victims.

Table 10.2 compares criminal predictors of the four outcomes under the headings of self-reports, convictions, and arrests. Similar to Table 10.1, all of the predictors of violent offenders were significant. However, in six cases (concerning robbery and aggravated assault), the predictor was logically related to the outcome; anyone who committed robbery or aggravated assault would inevitably be classified as a violent offender. Unlike Table 10.1, most of the criminal predictors of homicide offenders (50 out of 57, or 88%) were significant, as were 61% (35) of the predictors of homicide victims. However, only 40% (23) of the criminal predictors of shooting victims were significant, and most of the significant predictors (14) were based on self-reports. This suggests that the homicide offenders had the most versatile previous criminal history, while the shooting victims were the least versatile, with the homicide victims falling in between. The shooting victims had the least extensive criminal backgrounds. In contrast, the criminal backgrounds of the homicide victims, compared to the shooting victims, were much more distinct. It may be that the conflict between homicide offenders and homicide victims was more serious, culminating in eliminating a contestant or rival by means of a killing, whereas wounding may have reflected a less serious type of conflict (such as teaching someone a lesson).

Surprisingly, the criminal predictors of homicide offenders, homicide victims, and shooting victims were not significantly related. This was partly because of the low number (7) of nonsignificant predictors of homicide offenders. Of 50 significant criminal predictors of homicide offenders, 62% (31) were also significant criminal predictors of homicide victims, but so were 57% (4 out of 7) of the nonsignificant predictors of homicide offenders (OR = 1.2, CI = 0.2–6.1). Of 50 significant predictors of homicide offenders, 40% (20) were also significant predictors of shooting victims, but so were 43% (3 out of 7) of the nonsignificant predictors of homicide offenders (OR = 1.2, CI = 0.2–4.4).

The strongest relationship was between criminal predictors of homicide victims and shooting victims. Of 35 significant predictors of homicide victims, 46% (16) were also significant predictors of shooting victims, as were 32% (7) of the 22 nonsignificant predictors of homicide victims (OR = 1.8, CI = 0.6–5.5). Overall, the particular criminal predictors of one of these three outcomes did not significantly overlap with the criminal predictors of another.

Are predictors of homicide offenders qualitatively different from predictors of violent offenders? We found in Chap. 5 that, with one exception, the predictors of homicide offenders were also predictors of violence. In other words, there were no substantial qualitative differences between predictors of homicide offenders and violence. However, a larger percentage of homicide offenders, compared to violent offenders, were exposed to many of the risk factors. Thus differences between risk factors predicting homicide offenders and violent offenders were mostly of a quantitative rather than a qualitative nature.

Did homicide offenders, compared to homicide victims, grow up under more deprived conditions or were they exposed to more risk factors? The results showed that homicide offenders, compared to homicide victims, did not grow up more deprived or exposed to more risk factors. We found that homicide offenders were not more extreme than homicide victims on explanatory factors, with four factors predicting both groups: old for the grade (i.e., held back in school), lack of guilt, family on welfare, and broken home. However, the strongest predictors of homicide offenders were mostly socioeconomic factors: broken home, a bad neighborhood, the family on welfare, a young mother, and an unemployed mother. In contrast, the strongest predictors of homicide victims were mostly individual factors, such as lack of guilt and school problems (low academic achievement, old for the grade, and hyperactivity–impulsivity–attention deficit). Although both homicide offenders and homicide victims did not fare well in school, this was most obvious for homicide victims. As a result, both groups were cut off from further education and restricted in their employment in the regular economy. Instead, as mentioned, the two groups were engaged in several aspects of the black, illegal economy, as shown by their prior offenses such as receiving stolen goods.

Do early risk factors predict homicide offenders more accurately than homicide victims? A comparison of the integrated prediction exercises for each group (data on which Figs. 4.6 and 6.6 are based) shows AUCs of .870 for the prediction of homicide offenders and .840 for homicide victims. Thus, risk factors predicted homicide victims almost as well as homicide offenders.

Are homicide victims and shooting victims similar in their antisocial behavior? And, *Do early risk factors predict homicide victims more accurately than shooting victims?* The results showed much overlap between the predictors of homicide victims and shooting victims in each of the three domains: explanatory, behavioral, and criminal factors. Thus, many of the risk factors for homicide victims were also risk factors for shooting victims, and involved domains of the family, school and peers. However, the predictive efficacy as expressed in the AUC was lower for shooting victims than for homicide victims (.733 vs. .840). This may suggest the exposure to known risk factors was somewhat higher for homicide victims than for shooting victims.

To what extent do similar criminal offenses (and thus offense histories) predict violent offenders, homicide offenders, homicide victims, and shooting victims? Table 10.2 makes this comparison for self-reported delinquency, convictions, and arrests. The results show that there are more shared criminal predictors between homicide offenders and homicide victims than between homicide offenders and shooting victims. In both comparisons, homicide offenders were predicted by a larger array of criminal behaviors than either homicide victims or shooting victims, and this conclusion holds for self-reported delinquency, convictions, and arrests. Thus, homicide offenders were the most extreme on criminal predictors, followed by homicide victims, and then shooting victims. This pattern was observed across the categories of offenses (violence, property, drug, other). We will return to the topic of prior offense patterns when discussing theoretical explanations of homicide offenders and homicide victims.

   Are homicide offenders and victims similar in their antisocial behavior? The results from Chaps. 4–6 indicate that, in terms of prior self-reported delinquency, homicide offenders and homicide victims have engaged in a wide variety of delinquent acts. However, homicide victims, compared to homicide offenders, were slightly more likely to carry a gun, use a weapon or to be involved in gang fighting. In contrast, homicide offenders, compared to homicide victims, were more likely to have been a gang member and persistent drug user, to carry a weapon, and to have sold marijuana or hard drugs. Comparison of the findings for shooting victims and those who died showed that shooting victims and homicide victims engaged in a range of illicit behaviors, including selling hard drugs and marijuana and carrying a gun, which typically are associated with a high probability of interpersonal conflict, resulting in death for some.

Theoretical Aspects of the Development of Violence and Homicide Offending

In Chap. 1 we raised the question: *On the basis of the empirical findings, which criminological theories best explain the development of young homicide offenders and victims?* In general, developmental and life-course theories aim to explain the course of development of offending, the influence of risk factors, and the effect of life events (Farrington, 2005). Such theories can help to explain how and why biological factors such as a low heart rate, individual factors such as high impulsiveness or low intelligence, family factors such as poor parental supervision, peer factors, socioeconomic factors, and neighborhood factors influence the development of an individual potential for violence. As mentioned, homicide offending is an extreme form of violence. For example, living in a bad neighborhood and suffering socioeconomic deprivation may in some way cause poor parenting, which in some way causes high impulsiveness and school failure, which in some way causes a high potential for violence. Theories can also help in specifying more general concepts that underlie violence potential, such as low self-control or weak bonding to society. Theories can also help in specifying how a potentially violent person interacts with situational factors to produce violent acts, including homicide.

Figure 10.1 shows the key elements of the "Integrated Cognitive Antisocial Potential" (ICAP) theory (Farrington, 2003). It was designed to explain *offending* by lower class males and has been modified to explain the development of violence and homicide offending. It integrates ideas from many other theories, including strain, control, learning, labeling, and rational choice approaches; its key construct is antisocial potential (AP); and it assumes that the translation from antisocial potential to violent behavior depends on cognitive (thinking and decision-making) processes that take account of opportunities and victims. An independent test of the ICAP theory in the Netherlands by Van Der Laan, Blom, and Kleemans (2009) concluded that serious delinquency was related to an accumulation of long-term risk factors and also to situational factors such as using alcohol or drugs.

Figure 10.1 is deliberately simplified in order to show the key elements of the ICAP theory on one page; for example, it does not show how the processes operate differently for onset compared with desistance or at different ages. The key construct underlying offending is antisocial potential (AP), which refers to the potential to commit antisocial acts, including violence. Long-term persisting between-individual differences in AP are distinguished from short-term within-individual variations in AP. Long-term AP depends on impulsiveness, on strain, modeling and socialization processes, and on life events, while short-term variations in AP depend on motivating and situational factors. The ICAP theory suggests that long-term individual, family, peer, school, and neighborhood influences lead to the development of long-term, fairly stable, slowly changing differences between individuals in the potential for violence.

Regarding long-term AP, people can be ordered on a continuum from low to high. The distribution of AP in the population at any age is highly skewed; relatively few people have high levels of AP. People with high AP are more likely to commit many different types of antisocial acts including violence. Hence, offending and antisocial behavior are versatile rather than specialized. The relative ordering of people on AP (long-term between-individual variation) tends to be consistent over time, but absolute levels of AP vary with age, peaking in the teenage years, because of changes within individuals in the contextual factors that influence long-term AP (e.g., from childhood to adolescence, the increasing importance of peers and decreasing importance of parents).

Following strain theory, the main energizing factors that potentially lead to high long-term AP are desires for material goods, status among intimates, excitement,

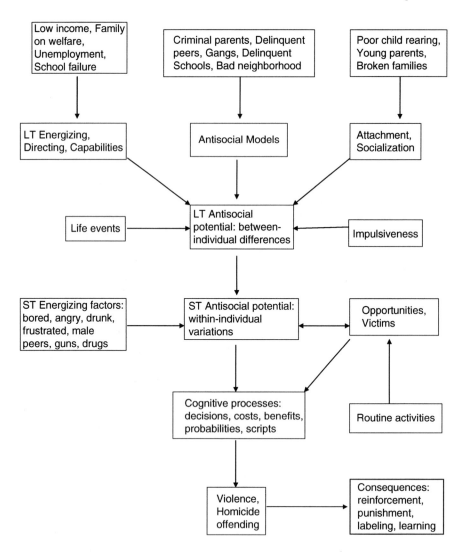

Note: LT = Long-Term; ST = Short-Term

Fig. 10.1 The integrated cognitive antisocial potential (ICAP) theory (Farrington, 2003)

and sexual satisfaction. However, these motivations only lead to high AP if antisocial methods of satisfying them are habitually chosen. Antisocial methods tend to be chosen by people who find it difficult to satisfy their needs legitimately, such as people with low income, families on welfare, unemployed people, and those who fail at school. However, the methods chosen also depend on physical capabilities and behavioral skills; for example, a 5-year-old would have difficulty stealing a car. For simplicity, energizing and directing processes and capabilities are shown in one box in Fig. 10.1.

Long-term AP also depends on attachment and socialization processes. AP will be low if parents consistently and contingently reward good behavior and punish bad behavior. (Withdrawal of love may be a more effective method of socialization than hitting children.) AP will be high if children are not attached to (prosocial) parents, for example, if parents are cold and rejecting. Broken families, which are often associated with young parents (Nagin, Pogarsky, & Farrington, 1997), may impair both attachment and socialization processes.

Long-term AP will also be high if people are exposed to and influenced by antisocial models, such as criminal parents, delinquent siblings, delinquent peers, and gangs in high crime schools and neighborhoods. Long-term AP will also be high for impulsive people, because they tend to act without thinking about the consequences, and for those with lack of guilt. Also, life events affect AP; it decreases after people get married or move out of high crime areas, and it increases after separation from a partner (see Farrington & West, 1995; Theobald & Farrington, 2009). There may also be interaction effects between the influences on long-term AP. For example, people who experience strain or poor socialization may be disproportionally antisocial if they are also exposed to antisocial models. In the interests of simplicity, Fig. 10.1 does not attempt to show such interactions.

According to the ICAP theory, the commission of offenses depends on the interaction between the individual (with his immediate level of AP) and the social environment (especially criminal opportunities and victims). Superimposed on long-term between-individual differences in violence potential are short-term within-individual variations. Short-term AP varies within individuals according to short-term energizing factors such as being bored, angry, drunk, or frustrated, being encouraged by male peers, and possession of guns or drugs. Criminal opportunities and the availability of victims depend on routine activities. Encountering a tempting opportunity or victim may cause a short-term increase in AP, just as a short-term increase in AP may motivate a person to seek out criminal opportunities and victims.

Faced with an opportunity for violence, whether a person with a certain level of AP actually is violent depends on cognitive processes, including considering the subjective benefits, costs and probabilities of the different outcomes and stored behavioral repertoires or scripts (based on previous experiences). The subjective benefits and costs include immediate situational factors such as the perceived utility of hurting someone and the likelihood and consequences of being caught by the police. They also include social factors such as likely disapproval by parents or female partners, and encouragement or reinforcement from peers (e.g., gang members). In general, people tend to make decisions that seem rational to them, but those with low levels of AP will not commit offenses even when (on the basis of subjective expected utilities) it appears rational to do so. Equally, high short-term levels of AP (e.g., caused by anger or drunkenness) may induce people to commit offenses when it is not rational for them to do so.

The consequences of violence may, as a result of a learning process, lead to changes in long-term AP and in future cognitive decision-making processes. This is especially likely if the consequences are reinforcing (e.g., gaining pleasure or peer approval) or punishing (e.g., receiving legal sanctions or parental disapproval). Also, if the consequences involve labeling or stigmatizing the offender, this may make it more difficult for him to achieve his aims legally, and hence may lead to an increase in AP. (It is difficult to show these feedback effects in Fig. 10.1 without making it very complex.) This kind of developmental theory might explain the development of violence and homicide offending and also suggest methods of intervention.

The ICAP theory can be modified to explain the development of homicide victims (and shooting victims). Most theories of homicide offending and victimization focus on immediate situation influences (e.g., routine activities, lifestyles, guns, gangs, and drugs) or neighborhood influences (e.g., social disorganization or concentrated disadvantage theories) (see e.g., MacDonald & Gover, 2005). Existing theories assume that homicide offenders and victims are similar in their lifestyles and in their neighborhood of residence, and this is why they come together in the homicide event.

In explaining the development of homicide victims, the top half in Fig. 10.1 of the ICAP theory would be unchanged. It would be assumed that most victims developed antisocial potential in the same way as offenders. However, the bottom half of Fig. 10.1, focusing on immediate situational influences and how antisocial potential was translated into a homicide victim, would change. In its simplest form, the theory would assume that long-term antisocial potential, short-term energizing factors (e.g., guns, gangs, drugs, arguments) and routine activities would influence the likelihood of a man becoming a homicide victim. Thus, the homicide victims would result from the interaction between antisocial potential and the immediate situational influences that tend to cause a homicide event.

According to this theory, both homicide offenders and most homicide victims would develop antisocial potential. However, the influences on victims could be somewhat different from the influences on homicide offenders. For example, in agreement with our results, it would be hypothesized that individual factors (e.g., impulsiveness and school failure) were more important for homicide victims, whereas socioeconomic factors (e.g., family on welfare, young parents, broken family, bad neighborhood) were more important for homicide offenders. It could also be hypothesized that homicide victims were less antisocial than homicide offenders, although our research suggests that they are quite similar in this respect.

Property Crime, Violence, and the Illegal Economy. In Chap. 1 we discussed the notion that what brought homicide offenders and homicide victims together was a cycle of conflict ("violence begets violence") and that this also seemed to apply to violent offenders and shooting victims. We also raised the possibility that what links offenders and their victims is engagement in various forms of property crime with the possibility of strong economic gains. Whereas drug dealing is often thought to be the key offense type in this respect, we found that several other illicit property activities, such trading stolen goods, car theft, and thefts of objects from cars, also contributed to homicidal and shooting victimization. Years ago, Sampson and Lauritsen (1990) using cross-sectional data from the British Crime Survey noted that those young males who were involved in vandalism and theft were at an increased risk of being assaulted. Rosenfeld (2009) proposed that acquisitive forms of crime drive the rate of violent crime, and demonstrated the secular covariation between acquisitive crime and homicide victimization. He argued that it is important to better understand the role of the underground economic markets in the causation of both property and violent crime.

Recently, Berg (2009) on the basis of new analyses of the PYS violence data demonstrated that the association between violent offending and victimization was geographically concentrated. Whereas the relationship between violent offending and victimization was virtually zero in advantaged neighborhoods, it was strong in the more disadvantaged neighborhoods. This accords with consistent evidence of the concentration of African American young men in the most disadvantaged neighborhoods, and agrees with the consistent finding of the critical nexus between the high rate of homicide and violent offending by African American young men and the high rate of African American young men becoming a homicide or a nonlethal shooting victim (discussed below more in detail). As mentioned in Chap. 3, most homicide events involved African American male offenders and African American male victims. Berg (2009) also documented the strong association between income-generating offending and victim status, showing that among the best predictors of violent victimization were marijuana and hard drug sales and illicit property transactions. When other covariates were introduced in a logistic regression, illicit property transactions survived in the analyses but not drug sales. This finding underscores the importance of engagement in the underground economy as a driving force for violence (and homicide) victimization.

In addition, we propose that illegal forms of property crime attract aggressive and impulsive young males (a selection effect) who are at risk of becoming homicide offenders, homicide victims, or both. Piquero and colleagues (Piquero, MacDonald, Dobrin, Daigle, & Cullen, 2005) presented evidence of a selection effect among homicide offenders and homicide victims, Using a 5-year follow-up of the records of postparole data the authors found that poor self-control was characteristic of both homicide offenders and homicide victims. Koolhof, Loeber, Wei, Pardini, and D'Escury (2007), using PYS data, found that low intelligent boys, compared to higher intelligent boys, exhibited the highest levels of cognitive and behavioral impulsivity. In addition, low intelligent boys were exposed to more risk factors for serious delinquency than higher intelligent boys, including living in a bad neighborhood. Lynam and colleagues (Lynam et al., 2000), also using PYS data, demonstrated that the effect of impulsivity on juvenile offending is stronger in the poorest compared to the more affluent neighborhoods. Thus, there appears to be a convergence of low intelligent, highly impulsive and aggressive young men in the most disadvantaged neighborhoods.

As articulated in Fig. 10.1, we hypothesize that broken families and poor parenting in the most disadvantaged neighborhoods and the high density of other risk factors in those areas creates a concentration of impulsive young males. From at least adolescence onward these impulsive young males, who often did poorly in school and whose employability over time became limited, are vying for economic resources outside of the customary forms of employment of legally sanctioned activities. We postulate that impulsive, low-self-controlled young males engaging in illegal property transactions generate conflicts with like-minded others. These two elements go together with nonreporting or underreporting of crime and victimization to the police (Berg, Slocum, & Loeber, 2011), and may lead to the administration of "personal justice" by contestants for money and power.

Race and Homicide Offenders and Homicide Victims

As mentioned in Chaps. 1 and 4–6, African American males compared to Caucasian males in this study, and in studies of violence and homicide elsewhere in the USA, are heavily overrepresented as homicide offenders, violent offenders, and as homicide and violence victims (Poe-Yamagata, & Jones, 2000; Pope & Snyder, 2003). The differential between the two racial groups was not always like this, but dramatically increased for African American homicide after 1985, peaked in 1994, and although lower subsequently has remained high since then (when compared to pre-1985 figures) (Berg, 2009). Thus, African American youth in the last two decades have increasingly been drawn into homicide offending and victimization.

African American boys were highly overrepresented among the homicide offenders in the PYS. We found that 32 out of the 37 homicide offenders were African American, as well as 439 out of the 652 other violent boys (two-thirds). In three chapters (Chaps. 4–6) we examined why this would be the case. We rejected the idea that higher homicide offending and violence by African American young males was inherently related to their race. In the present study, we could not address decision makers' bias as a potential source for the disproportionate representation of African American young males in the justice system (Poe-Yamagata & Jones, 2000; Pope & Snyder, 2003). Instead, we proposed that the racial difference is at least partly observed because African American young males, compared to their Caucasian counterparts, are exposed to more known risk factors for violence manifest in disadvantaged neighborhoods with their associated problems of concentrated poverty and other social ills. Thus the question we raised is: *Are racial differences in the prevalence of violent and homicide offenders, homicide victims and shooting victims attributable to racial differences in early risk factors?* We answered this question by means of logistic regression analyses to establish whether race was an independent predictor of homicide and violence once other risk factors were known and taken into account. The results were as follows. Chapter 4 showed that, after the nine best explanatory predictors of homicide were entered into the equation, African American race was no longer a significant predictor of homicide offending. The best explanatory predictors were a broken family, living in a bad neighborhood, the family on welfare, a young mother, old for the grade (held back in school), an unemployed mother, lack of guilt, behavior problems of the father, and low socioeconomic status. Thus, many aspects of social disadvantage and not race predicted future homicide offenders.

We repeated the analyses in Chap. 5 for violence, and for the prediction of homicide offenders out of the violent offenders. African American race significantly predicted violence, but we did not find that African American race independently predicted homicide offenders out of the violent offenders once other risk factors were taken into account. Only when homicide arrestees were combined with homicide offenders, did African American race contribute to the prediction (Table 5.4). This may reflect the higher arrest rate of African American young males, compared with Caucasian males, that is evident from many studies (e.g., Fite, Wynn, & Pardini, 2009; Heide, 2003). It may be that African American males are more likely to be arrested when they are in fact innocent. Fite, Wynn, and Pardini (2009) investigated disproportionate minority arrest in the PYS, and found that a higher incidence of risk factors accounted for racial differences related to any type of juvenile arrest, as well as differences in violence- and theft-related arrest, but not drug-related arrests.

Earlier analyses in the PYS on the prediction of violence found that African American status did not independently predict violence (Farrington, Loeber, & Stouthamer-Loeber, 2003; Loeber et al., 2005a). Later analyses using data as well from the Denver Youth Study and the Rochester Youth Development Study (Huizinga et al., 2006) confirmed that, in the majority of prediction analyses, African American race did not independently contribute to the prediction of violence once other risk factors were known. Also, recent analyses on violence in different age ranges of the PYS, showed that, even though African American race predicted violence in three developmental periods, it did not contribute to the prediction of violence in any of the seven logistic regressions (Loeber et al., 2008). Thus, the analyses mostly agree that the correlation between African American race and later violence is mediated by a host of risk factors.

Another test of race as a possible explanation of homicide is to determine the extent to which race predicts homicide victims and shooting victims. Results presented in Chap. 6 show that, after 11 significant explanatory risk factors were entered in a logistic regression analysis, race was still a significant predictor of homicide victims. This may primarily be because 37 of the 39 homicide victims were African American. Similar results were obtained for shooting victims, but the predictive power of race was considerably reduced after controlling for explanatory risk factors. We conclude that much of the relationship between race and homicide offenders and shooting victims is explained by racial differences in risk factors, but the evidence is less strong for homicide victims.

In summary, known risk factors for violence (and homicide offending) account for racial disparities in homicide and violent offending and victimization. It is likely that African Americans' exposure to risk factors in their physical and social environments rather than their race, explains why some African American males show problem behaviors and/or violence (see also Haynie & Armstrong, 2006; Wilson, Hurtt, Shaw, Dishion, & Gardner, 2009). In the PYS, the most important of these risk factors were broken home, the family on welfare, a bad neighborhood, and a young mother.

Screening and Risk/Needs Assessment

In Chap. 1 we raised the following questions pertaining to screening:

- *To what extent is it possible to develop and use a screening instrument to predict persons who are at risk of becoming homicide offenders or victims?*
- *Is a step-wise screen more efficient in the prediction of homicide offenders compared to a single screen?*
- *Is it possible to model screening and establish whether an early screen is more efficient in identifying homicide offenders than a screen administered at a later age?*
- *Is a screening instrument for the prediction of homicide offenders better or worse than a screening instrument for the prediction of homicide victims?*

Our results on the prediction of homicide offenders and homicide victims show that many risk factors are important predictors. Among the independent explanatory risk factors are broken home, a bad neighborhood, the family on welfare, low SES, an unemployed mother, a young mother, large family size, hyperactivity–impulsivity–attention deficit, low school achievement, lack of guilt, and callous-unemotional behavior. Among the independent behavioral (and attitudinal) risk factors are suspended from school, truant, low school motivation, Disruptive Behavior Disorder, an antisocial attitude, delinquent peers, and many prior arrests, especially for offenses such as receiving stolen property, vehicle theft, drugs, assault, and weapons.

When these items were combined into risk scales, it was possible to identify a high-risk group of about 15–20% of the sample, of whom 8–14% became convicted homicide offenders, including at least half of all homicide offenders. However, the boys in the PYS are themselves a relatively high-risk group, since they were selected after the application of a screening risk assessment. Therefore, it seems realistic to suggest that, in real life prospective use in communities, a high-risk group identified by a risk assessment instrument might include 5–10% who are convicted for homicide and 5–10% who are killed, in turn perhaps identifying 40–50% of all homicide offenders and victims. Therefore, the false-positive rate would be high (90–95%). This rate could be reduced by applying the instrument to persons identified as high risk (e.g., because of offending).

In the interests of reducing the false-positive rate, we suggest that two screening instruments might be developed and tested, based on our results: one applied at age 7–8 to predict violence, and one applied at age 13–14 to predict homicide offenders and victims. The age 7–8 assessment might be applied in schools or to children who are referred for problematic behavior, building on the EARL-20B (Augimeri, Koegl, Webster, & Levene, 2001), which includes many of the risk factors that we have identified. The age 13–14 assessment might be applied to arrested children, building on the SAVRY (Borum, Bartel, & Forth, 2006). Any instrument would need to be designed for ease of use by practitioners, for example, requiring scoring on only about 20 risk factors. It is also important for instruments to assess needs as well as risk, so that children's needs can be addressed in treatment programs, which should be designed to help children and families, not punish them. It is also important to avoid stigmatizing children and families.

Justice Response: Incarceration and Waiver to Adult Court

This volume did not explicitly deal with the criminal careers of homicide offenders in the juvenile and adult courts. Six homicide offenders were convicted of first-degree murder, six of second-degree murder, and 17 of third-degree murder. There were three convictions for manslaughter, one for conspiracy to commit homicide, one for vehicular homicide, and one for a homicide of unknown degree. Two offenders were not sentenced because they were killed. Sentence length varied: 12 offenders were sentenced to life imprisonment, and 3 of these were sentenced to life without parole. Since their sentence, this has been declared illegal. Of the remaining homicide offenders, 13 were sentenced to more than 10 years, and 5 of these to more than 20 years. Five offenders received sentences of less than 5 years. Invariably, if a homicide offender was convicted when below age 18, his case was automatically transferred to the adult court.

In summary, the commission of homicide followed by a court trial and conviction was a turning point in the lives of the young men who killed. For those who were found guilty this meant losing their freedom, adapting to prison life, curtailing their noncriminal professional careers, losing caring fatherhood and intimate partnerships, and, for a proportion of the adolescent young men, doing time with adult offenders.

For society, violence and homicide come at a high cost: the loss of life and the loss of income generated by the victim for his dependents, the trauma for the relatives and friends of the victim, the costs of emergency and hospital care before the victim died, and last but not least, the cost of incarceration of homicide offenders over years to come. For example, in 2006 three quarters of a million young people between ages 10 and 24 were treated in emergency rooms for assault-related injuries (Foreman, 2009), which must constitute a huge expense. A report on violence (including self-inflicted violence) and health care showed that in Pennsylvania in 1994 just over 90,000 individuals were seen in an emergency department because of an injury caused by violence. Just under a quarter of these injury cases required hospitalization with the cost of the admissions amounting to $233 million. Out of the hospital admissions for violence about one in ten died (Highmark, 2000). Thus, the number of homicides is dwarfed by the incidence of violence that does not lead to death. The average cost of a hospital stay was $6,582 for interpersonal violence at the time of the study. The burden that community violence puts on hospitals is very large, and its costs are eventually carried by taxpayers.

The cost of incarceration is also high: in 2008, the average annual cost of incarceration for Federal inmates was $25,895, and for an inmate in a Community Corrections Center it was $23,882 (http://edocket.access.gpo.gov/2009/E9-16304.htm, accessed

17 July 2010). For a 20-year-old inmate to serve life in a Federal prison of, say, 40 years, this would cost over one million dollars ($1,035,800).[3]

It can be argued that retribution by means of a long sentence is a just desert for as hideous a crime as homicide. However, it is debatable who is best served in this respect: certainly not the victim, perhaps satisfied relatives, but the costs to society are huge. This is why we discussed preventive interventions in Chaps. 8 and 9.

Preventive Interventions

Earlier in this chapter, we made a case that there is a chain of causes that unfolds over time and leads to homicide offending in some young males. We argue that there is a need to undertake preventive interventions early in that chain rather than at a later point. However, it can be argued that perhaps homicide offenders emerge in society because of failed services. Stouthamer-Loeber et al. (2001a), using an early version of the PYS homicide data set ($N = 29$ homicide offenders), examined whether homicide offenders compared to violent offenders used more mental health services (defined as any help sought for a child's mental health problems, which included not only professional help) or school services (consisting of mainly special education services and classes for behavior problems). The results show that two-thirds of the homicide offenders when young had received help for behavior problems, which was significantly higher than other violent offenders. In terms of school services, the authors did not find a difference between the two groups. Thus, despite the fact that homicide offenders tended to receive a variety of services for their behavior and mental problems, the interventions apparently failed to stop these young men in their progress to homicide offending. Unfortunately, it proved impossible to gauge the exact nature of the services and to assess their quality and whether they were based on empirically verified interventions, which, in hindsight, appears debatable.

We argue that empirical knowledge about what works and knowledge of the causes of homicide offending and violence is essential in helping to determine the optimal timing and effectiveness of preventive interventions, and in providing the basis for screening people for their risk of killing or getting killed, which is an area that is poorly developed (Hardwick & Rowton-Lee, 1996). The U.S. Surgeon General called for a reduction in homicide victimization (in all age groups) from 6.5 deaths per 100,000 person-years in 1998 to less than 3.0 deaths per 100,000 person-years in 2010 (U.S. Department of Health and Human Services, 2000), but it remains to be seen whether this goal is attainable, and if attainable whether factors that cause such a decrease are understood. The latter point is debatable, because there is a wide-spread lack of knowledge about processes leading up to homicide offending. It is precisely this knowledge that is vital for improving public safety and reducing

---

[3] Note that slightly lower costs have been mentioned in Chap. 8, which was based on earlier figures.

the risk of homicide offending in the general population, but particularly in the highest risk groups of adolescent and young adult males. To address these important issues, this volume contains two modeling studies that assess the potential effect of interventions on reducing the rate of homicide.

In Chap. 8 we stressed that the absence of homicide as an outcome in known experimental interventions is clearly related to the low prevalence of homicide among the small numbers of participants in quasi-experimental and randomized experimental studies. Also, many intervention studies with intermediate outcomes such as aggression and violence have a limited number of years of follow-up, a point which is important because of the relatively long latency time and relative rarity of homicide offending (and homicide victimization). We argued that, for these reasons alone, it is useful to simulate (or model) the impact of interventions by using existing longitudinal data. In Chap. 8 we focused on the modeling of interventions on a national scale, whereas in Chap. 9 we focused on interventions on a local level. Both chapters address the question "what if…" we changed one aspect of individuals' problem behavior, what impact does that have on future homicide and violent offending?

Chapter 8 shows a modeling exercise to demonstrate the impact of selected interventions implemented nationally on the male national homicide rate in urban and nonurban populations. The modeling used data from the youngest and oldest PYS cohorts and was based on the sequential implementation of three well-evaluated early preventive interventions for at-risk populations of youth and their families: the Olds Nurse Home Visitation Program, the Perry Preschool Program, and multisystemic therapy (MST) for juvenile violent offenders (see Fig. 8.1). The following are the most salient results:

- Nationwide implementation of the Nurse Home Visitation Program by itself with at-risk families is projected to prevent one-fifth (21.7%) of all homicides in the USA, with 50,000 person-years of victims' potential life saved annually. This strategy alone has the potential to reduce the cost of incarceration by about $3.5 billion.
- Nationwide implementation of the Perry Preschool Program for preschoolers could potentially also reduce homicides by up to one quarter (24%), saving annually just over 3,000 lives, resulting in almost $4 billion savings in incarceration costs.
- Nationwide implementation of MST for juvenile delinquents by itself would have a lower effect on homicide (a reduction of 6% annually), nevertheless resulting in almost $800 million savings in incarceration cost.

The sequential implementation of the three programs for different ages of youth produced in even better results: reducing homicide offending by a third (33%), saving 4,205 lives annually and resulting in more than a $5 billion reduction in the costs of incarceration. It should be kept in mind that Chap. 8 also provides details of the impact of these striking results, showing the relatively high confidence intervals. On the other hand, the results would be stronger if nonhomicidal violence also had been taken into account.

Violence and homicide offending are addressed in the second modeling exercise, also based on the PYS (Chap. 9), but with the aim of modeling the impact of interventions on local homicides, arrest for violence, and cost of incarceration. We focused on two at-risk populations. The first at-risk population consisted of young boys with the worst disruptive/delinquent behavior at the beginning of the PYS, who were identified by means of a screening risk index (based on youth self-reports, and parent- and teacher-ratings). The second at-risk population consisted of those youth arrested for violence (recorded usually at a later age than the risk index). For each risk group we assumed an intervention with a success rate of 30% (based on the effect sizes of optimal interventions available from the intervention research literature). In a variant on the earlier modeling exercise presented in Chap. 8, Chap. 9 focused on cumulative changes in behavior over years. Specifically, we were interested in the lowering of the age–crime curve, and of the arrest rate for nonhomicidal violence, homicide offenders, and homicide victims. In addition we were keen to express the impact of interventions in terms of the dollars saved because of the reduced cost of incarceration.

The first screen at the beginning of the study identified 772 high-risk cases from the three cohorts ($N = 1,517$), of which we selected the upper 30% for the intervention ($N = 232$). Without any intervention, the age–crime curve of arrests represented almost two-and-a-half thousand arrests for violence. The intervention at an early age, especially before age 13, lowered the age–crime curve of arrests for violence by 20% (482 fewer arrests). In addition, the intervention lowered the number of homicide offenders by 30%, and reduced the number of weeks of incarceration by one-fifth (21.7%), which translates into a reduction of incarceration by over 100 person-years (107.7). Thus, there were substantial gains and savings as a result of the modeling of an intervention with a success rate of 30%.

The second intervention (also with an assumed success rate of 30%) followed the first intervention for youth who despite the first intervention had been arrested for violence at age 14, which means an early-onset group of serious delinquents. The implementation of the first and second interventions in sequence, especially after age 14, further lowered the age–crime curve of arrests for violence, but not noticeably for the age period 22–25. Also, the age–crime curve of arrests for violence as a result of the sequential implementation of the first and second interventions was only marginally lower than the age–crime curve for the first intervention only. Thus, the yield of the second intervention following the first was not substantial. This was also true for the reduction in homicide victims, but not for homicide offenders which were substantially reduced (40% vs. 30%). Moreover, the sequential application of the two interventions reduced the number of weeks of incarceration by 30%, compared to 22% for first intervention alone. We also examined the yield of the second intervention by itself, which showed that the first intervention, which focused on disruptive/delinquent youth at a young age, outperformed the second intervention by a high degree. The results also show that interventions have benefits that extend well beyond violence and extend to other forms of serious offending as well.

In summary, the model of interventions at a young age has higher yields in both modeling studies than the model of interventions at a later age. In addition, early interventions have the additional benefit of curtailing what otherwise might be years of violent victimization of others and years of commission of serious property crime. We argue that an intervention at a young age, compared to an intervention at a later age, reduces more offenders, victims, and offenses.

We also saw that the modeling studies show the additional yield of implementing successive interventions for different risk groups of youth, such as violent arrestees, as they become manifest over time. Both studies show substantial reductions in incarceration time and the financial costs attached to incarceration.

Our focus in the modeling exercises has been on high-risk populations. If screening at a young age is not feasible or too costly, it may be useful to focus a program on high-risk areas; not necessarily in the areas of the highest homicide rates or highest rates of assault with weapon, but in areas where there is the highest density of risk factors for future violence and homicide. This is a feature of the Communities That Care program, described below.

Pittsburgh as a Microcosm of Homicides, Violence, and Cries for Help

In Chap. 3 we showed that homicides in Pittsburgh have many characteristics in common with homicides in other major cities. The killings continue intermittently but predictably in Pittsburgh. The dismay and fear of citizens (see, e.g., the testimony in Chap. 1) periodically reaches the media to fade away subsequently (see also, Wideman, 2005). The city government, after long delays, is implementing a gang suppression program. Testimonies at public meetings also called for preventive early interventions (e.g., Coalition Against Violence, 2008). However, often community initiatives, dependent on the availability and laudable energy of local leaders, have relatively short lives. Efforts to implement "evidence-based interventions" in the absence of accountability and knowledge of empirical studies are easily overshadowed by calls for "logical," nontraditional and unevaluated programs. Calls for a concerted effort to prevent violence have been rare (e.g., How violence is eroding our quality of life, 2009). Mediation techniques are being implemented to reduce violence among warring parties. However, minors' access to and use of guns remains a persistent problem in the Pittsburgh community, and there is little sign of effective programs to reduce juveniles' access to firearms.

The role of the media in Pittsburgh is tremendously important. Whereas the infrequent murders (multiple or with children as victims) are reported well, daily systemic violence, and typical homicides are underreported. Since violent offenders comprise the reservoir from which homicide offenders eventually emerge, it would be very helpful if the media would focus more on interpersonal violence in the community. Only then, the frequent reminders can help communities to mount interventions to combat violence and homicide in particular.

Aside from conducting longitudinal studies, we have been successful in collaboration with an advisory panel of concerned community leaders to implement in two sites the *SNAP™ Program* for youth below age 12 exhibiting conduct problems and delinquent behavior (Hrynkiw-Augimeri, Pepler, & Goldberg, 1993; Pepler, Smith, & Rigby, 2004). Evaluation research shows that the *SNAP™ Program* (Augimeri, Farrington, Koegl, & Day, 2007; Koegl, Farrington, Augimeri, & Day, 2008), compared to controls produced significant reductions in child problem behavior. Currently, the program is being evaluated in a randomized controlled design.

Policy Implications for National and Local Initiatives

In Chap. 1 we asked: *How can current policies to reduce youth violence and homicide offending be optimized?* Intervention programs to reduce violence and homicide offending should be based on knowledge about risk and protective factors (Farrington, 2001b, 2007b). More systematic reviews and meta-analyses of these factors are needed, and more randomized experiments should be mounted to evaluate the effectiveness of risk-focused prevention. High quality evaluation research shows that many types of programs are effective, and that in many cases their financial benefits outweigh their financial costs (Farrington & Welsh, 2007). However, there have been relatively few attempts to study effects on violence specifically (and no attempts to study effects on homicide offending) or to follow up experimental and control individuals in repeated interviews (see Farrington, 2006). Also, there are few intervention programs targeted on homicide victims.

The major policy implications are as follows: Impulsiveness should be targeted by skills training (Lösel & Beelmann, 2006), and low school achievement should be targeted by preschool intellectual enrichment programs (Schweinhart et al., 2005). Smoking, drinking, and drug use in pregnancy, and early child abuse, should be targeted by home visiting programs in which nurses give advice to mothers about prenatal and postnatal care of the child, about infant development, and about the importance of proper nutrition and avoiding substance use in pregnancy (Olds, Sadler, & Kitzman, 2007). Poor parental supervision and inconsistent discipline should be targeted by behavioral parent management training (Webster-Stratton, 1998). Negative peer influence should be a focus of community-based mentoring programs (Jolliffe & Farrington, 2008) and by treatment foster care (Chamberlain & Reid, 1998). Programs designed to encourage stable relationships and discourage early pregnancy and early motherhood should be mounted (Theobald & Farrington, 2010).

In addition, community programs that encourage cohesiveness, collective efficacy, and intervention to prevent crimes can also be recommended. "Communities That Care" (CTC) is one of the most promising community-based prevention programs (Hawkins & Catalano, 1992). It is modeled on large-scale community-wide public health programs, and it is a multiple-component program including interventions that have been proved to be effective in high quality research. It is based on the Seattle Social Development Project and the Social Development Model. The choice of intervention strategies depends on empirical evidence about what are the most important risk and protective factors in a particular community. The interventions aim to reduce the identified risk factors and enhance the identified protective factors. CTC has been shown to be effective in reducing substance use and delinquency in a large randomized experiment involving 24 communities (Hawkins et al., 2009). It should be implemented more widely in an effort to reduce violence and homicide offending.

It is also important to target immediate situational influences on violence such as alcohol, guns, gangs, and drugs. For example, the gang prevention program GREAT (Gang Resistance Education and Training) reduced victimization, instilled more negative views about gangs among youth, improved attitudes toward police, and increased the number of prosocial peers (Howell, 2009, p. 161). However, it did not prevent youth joining gangs. As another example, Macintyre and Homel (1997) in Australia found that violence in nightclubs was caused by crowding as well as drunkenness. They made recommendations about how nightclubs could be redesigned to reduce crowding, by changing pedestrian flow patterns (e.g., to and from restrooms). Following the ICAP theory, it would also be desirable to try to change decision-making by potential offenders in criminal opportunities, by decreasing subjectively perceived benefits and increasing subjectively perceived costs of violence.

The time is ripe to adopt a public health approach and embark on risk-focused prevention on a large scale, perhaps based on "Communities That Care," in order to reduce violence and homicide offending. This approach would have many additional benefits, including improving mental and physical health and life success in areas such as education, employment, relationships, housing, and childrearing. Obviously, any program that reduces homicide offenders would also reduce homicide victims. It is crucial to interrupt the intergenerational transmission of crime and violence, and the financial benefits of risk-focused prevention seem very likely to exceed the financial costs. We anticipate that risk-focused prevention, based on the risk factors identified in this book and based on proven interventions, could lead to significant reductions in violence and homicide offending.

References

Achenbach, T. M., & Edelbrock, C. S. (1979). The child behavior profile. II. Boys aged 12–16 and girls aged 6–11 and 12–16. *Journal of Consulting and Clinical Psychology, 47*, 223–233.

Achenbach, T. M., & Edelbrock, C. S. (1983). *Manual for the child behavior checklist and revised child behavior profile*. Burlington, VT: University of Vermont Department of Psychiatry.

Achenbach, T. M., & Edelbrock, C. S. (1987). *Manual for the youth self-report and profile*. Burlington, VT: University of Vermont Department of Psychiatry.

American Psychiatric Association. (1994). *Diagnostic and statistical manual of mental disorders (DSM-IV)*. Washington, DC: American Psychiatric Association.

Anderson, R. N., & Smith, B. L. (2002). Deaths: Leading causes for 2002. *National Vital Statistics Report, 53*, 1–92.

Angold, A., Erkanli, A., Loeber, R., Costello, E. J., Van Kammen, W., & Stouthamer-Loeber, M. (1996). Disappearing depression in a population of boys. *Journal of Emotional and Behavioral Disorders, 4*, 95–104.

Aos, S., Lieb, R., Mayfield, J., Miller, M., & Pennucci, A. (2004). *Benefits and costs of prevention and early intervention programs for youth*. Olympia, WA: Washington State Institute for Public Policy.

Arias, E., Anderson, R. N., Kung, H. C., Murphy, S. L., & Kochanek, K. D. (2003). Deaths: Final data for 2001. *National Vital Statistics Report, 52*, 1–115.

Augimeri, L. K., Farrington, D. P., Koegl, C. J., & Day, D. M. (2007). The under 12 outreach project: Effects of a community based program for children with conduct problems. *Journal of Child and Family Studies, 16*, 799–807.

Augimeri, L. K., Koegl, C. J., Webster, C. D., & Levene, K. S. (2001). *Early assessment risk list for boys (EARL-20B), version 2*. Toronto: Earlscourt Child and Family Centre.

Bailey, S. (1996). Adolescents that murder. *Journal of Adolescence, 19*, 19–39.

Barnoski, R. (2004). *Outcome evaluation of Washington state's research-based programs for juvenile offenders*. Olympia, WA: Washington State Institute for Public Policy.

Bender, L. (1959). Children and adolescents who have killed. *The American Journal of Psychiatry, 166*, 410–413.

Benedek, E. P., & Cornell, D. G. (1989). *Juvenile homicide*. Washington, DC: American Psychiatric Press.

Berg, M. T. (2009). *Understanding the persistence of the victimization-offending relationship: Modeling causal mechanisms across place and time*. Unpublished Ph.D. dissertation, University of Missouri, St. Louis, MO.

Berg, M. T., Slocum, L. A., & Loeber, R. (2011). Illegal behavior and police reporting by victims of violence. *Under review Journal of Quantitative Criminology*.

R. Loeber and D.P. Farrington, *Young Homicide Offenders and Victims*,
Longitudinal Research in the Social and Behavioral Sciences: An Interdisciplinary Series,
DOI 10.1007/978-1-4419-9949-8, © Springer Science+Business Media, LLC 2011

Beyers, J. M., Loeber, R., Wikström, P.-O. H., & Stouthamer-Loeber, M. (2001). What predicts adolescent violence in better-off neighborhoods? *Journal of Abnormal Child Psychology, 29*, 369–381.

Bijleveld, C., & Smit, P. (2006). Homicide in the Netherlands: On the structuring of homicide typologies. *Homicide Studies, 10*, 195–216.

Block, C. R., & Block, R. L. (2008, November). *Homicides connected to other homicides. An examination of the Chicago Homicide Dataset, 1965–2000.* Paper presented at the meeting of the American Society of Criminology, Washington, DC.

Blumstein, A., Rivara, F. P., & Rosenfeld, R. (2000). The rise and decline of homicide–and why. *Annual Review of Public Health, 21*, 505–541.

Blumstein, A., & Wallman, J. (2000). *The crime drop in America.* New York, NY: Cambridge University Press.

Blumstein, A., & Wallman, J. (Eds.). (2006). *The crime drop in America.* Cambridge: Cambridge University Press.

Borduin, C. M., Mann, B. J., Cone, L. T., Henggeler, S. W., Fucci, B. R., Blaske, D. M., et al. (1995). Multisystemic treatment of serious juvenile offenders: Long-term prevention of criminality and violence. *Journal of Consulting and Clinical Psychology, 63*, 569–578.

Borum, R., Bartel, P., & Forth, A. (2006). *Manual for the structured assessment of violence risk in youth (SAVRY).* Odessa, FL: Psychological Assessment Resources.

Braga, A. A. (2008). Pulling levers focused deterrence strategies and the prevention of gun homicide. *Journal of Criminal Justice, 36*, 332–343.

Brodie, L. M., Daday, J. K., Crandall, C. S., Sklar, D. P., & Jost, P. F. (2006). Exploring demographic, structural, and behavioral overlap among homicide offenders and victims. *Homicide Studies, 10*, 155–180.

Broidy, L. M., Nagin, D. S., Tremblay, R. E., Bates, J. E., Brame, B., Dodge, K. A., et al. (2003). Developmental trajectories of childhood disruptive behaviors and adolescent delinquency: A six-site, cross-national study. *Developmental Psychology, 39*, 222–245.

Brookman, F. (2005). *Understanding homicide.* London: Sage.

Bureau of Justice Statistics (2004a). *Expenditure and employment statistics.* Accessed August 17, from http://www.ojp.usdoj.gov/bjs/eande.htm.

Bureau of Justice Statistics (2004b). *Personal and property crimes, 2002: Total economic loss to victims of crime, national criminal victimization survey 2002.* Accessed August 17, from http://www.ojp.usdoj.gov/bjs/pub/pdf/cvus/current/cv0282.pdf.

Burgess, E. W. (1928). Factors determining success or failure on parole. In A. A. Bruce, A. J. Harno, E. W. Burgess, & J. Landesco (Eds.), *The workings of the indeterminate-sentence law and the parole system in Illinois* (pp. 205–249). Springfield, IL: Illinois State Board of Parole.

Busch, K. G., Zagar, R., Hughes, J. R., Arbit, J., & Bussell, R. E. (1990). Adolescents who kill. *Journal of Clinical Psychology, 46*, 472–485.

Campbell, D. T., & Stanley, J. C. (1966). *Experimental and quasi-experimental designs for research.* Chicago: Rand McNally.

Catalano, R. F., Arthur, M. W., Hawkins, J. D., Berglund, L., & Olson, J. J. (1998). Comprehensive community- and school-based interventions to prevent antisocial behavior. In R. Loeber & D. P. Farrington (Eds.), *Serious and violent juvenile offenders: Risk factors and successful interventions* (pp. 248–283). Thousand Oaks, CA: Sage.

Centers for Disease Control (2008, Summer). *Youth violence. Facts at a glance.* Atlanta, GA: Center for Disease Control. Accessed from http://www.cdc.gov/injury.

Centers for Disease Control and Prevention (2006). *WISQARS (Web-based Injury statistics query and reporting system).* Accessed January 3, from http://www.cdc.gov/ncipc/wisqars/.

Chamberlain, P., & Reid, J. B. (1998). Comparison of two community alternatives to incarceration for chronic juvenile offenders. *Journal of Consulting and Clinical Psychology, 66*, 624–633.

City of Pittsburgh Bureau of Police (2002). Statistical report.

Coalition Against Violence (2008, July 8). Meeting at Duquesne University, Pittsburgh.

Committee on Improving Evaluation of Anti-Crime Programs. (2005). *Improving evaluation of anticrime programs.* Washington, DC: National Academies Press.

Conroy, M., & Murrie, D. (2007). *Forensic assessment of violence risk: A guide for risk assessment and risk management*. Hoboken, NJ: Wiley.

Cook, P. J., & Laub, J. H. (1998). The unprecedented epidemic in youth violence. In M. Tonry & M. H. Moore (Eds.), *Youth violence* (pp. 27–64). Chicago: University of Chicago Press.

Cook, P. J., Ludwig, J., & Braga, A. A. (2005). Criminal records of homicide offenders. *Journal of the American Medical Association, 294*, 598–601.

Cornell, D. G., Benedek, E. P., & Benedek, D. M. (1987). Youth homicide: Prior adjustment and a proposed typology. *The American Journal of Orthopsychiatry, 57*, 383–392.

Costantino, J. P., Kuller, L. H., Perper, J. A., & Cypess, R. H. (1977). An epidemiologic study of homicides in Allegheny County, Pennsylvania. *American Journal of Epidemiology, 106*, 314–324.

Costello, E. J., Edelbrock, C., & Costello, A. J. (1985). The validity of the NIMH diagnostic interview schedule for children (DISC): A comparison between pediatric and psychiatric referrals. *Journal of Abnormal Child Psychology, 13*, 579–595.

Costello, A., Edelbrock, C. S., Kalas, R., Kessler, R., & Klaric, S. H. (1982). *The diagnostic interview schedule for children, parent version (revised)*. Worcester, MA: University of Massachusetts Medical Center.

Dalton, E., Yonas, M., Warren, L., & Sturman, E. (2009). *Research report: Violence in Allegheny County and Pittsburgh*. Pittsburgh: Allegheny County Department of Health. Unpublished report.

Decker, S. H. (1996). Deviant homicide: A new look at the role of motives and victim-offender relationships. *Journal of Research in Crime and Delinquency, 33*, 427–449.

Dobrin, A. (2001). The risk of offending in homicide victimization: A case control study. *Journal of Research in Crime and Delinquency, 38*, 154–173.

Edelbrock, C., & Achenbach, T. (1984). The teacher version of the Child Behavior Profile: I. Boys aged six through eleven. *Journal of Consulting and Clinical Psychology, 52*, 207–217.

Elliott, D. S., Huizinga, D., & Ageton, S. S. (1985). *Explaining delinquency and drug use*. Beverly Hills: Sage.

Epstein, R. M. (2006). Making communication research matter: What do patients notice, what do patients want, and what do patients need? *Patient Education and Counseling, 60*, 272–278.

Ezell, M. E., & Tanner-Smith, E. E. (2009). Examining the role of lifestyle and criminal history variables on the risk of homicide victimization. *Homicide Studies, 13*, 144–173.

Fabio, A., Cohen, J., & Loeber, R. (in press). Neighborhood socioeconomic disadvantage and the shape of the age-crime curve. *American Journal of Public Health*, in press.

Farrington, D. P. (1986). Age and crime. In M. Tonry, & N. Morris (Eds.), *Crime and justice* (Vol. 7, pp. 189–250). Chicago: University of Chicago Press.

Farrington, D. P. (1986). Age and crime. In M. Tonry, & N. Norris (Eds.), *Crime and justice: An annual review of research* (Vol. 7, pp. 189–250). Chicago: University of Chicago Press.

Farrington, D. P. (1991). Childhood aggression and adult violence: Early precursors and later life outcomes. In D. J. Pepler & K. H. Rubin (Eds.), *The development and treatment of childhood aggression* (pp. 8–30). Hillsdale, NJ: Erlbaum.

Farrington, D. P. (1996). *Understanding and preventing youth crime*. York, England: Joseph Rowntree Foundation.

Farrington, D. P. (1998). Predictors, causes, and correlates of male youth violence. In M. Tonry & M. H. Moore (Eds.), *Youth violence* (pp. 421–475). Chicago: University of Chicago Press.

Farrington, D. P. (2001a). Predicting adult official and self-reported violence. In G.-F. Pinard & L. Pagani (Eds.), *Clinical assessment of dangerousness: Empirical contributions* (pp. 66–88). Cambridge: Cambridge University Press.

Farrington, D. P. (2001b). The causes and prevention of violence. In J. Shepherd (Ed.), *Violence in health care* (2nd ed., pp. 1–27). Oxford: Oxford University Press.

Farrington, D. P. (2003). Developmental and life-course criminology: Key theoretical and empirical issues. *Criminology, 41*, 221–255.

Farrington, D. P. (Ed.). (2005). *Integrated developmental and life-course theories of offending (Advances in Criminological Theory, Vol. 14)*. New Brunswick, NJ: Transaction.

Farrington, D. P. (2006). Key longitudinal-experimental studies in criminology. *Journal of Experimental Criminology, 2*, 121–141.

Farrington, D. P. (2007a). Childhood risk factors and risk-focused prevention. In M. Maguire, R. Morgan, & R. Reiner (Eds.), *The Oxford handbook of criminology* (4th ed., pp. 602–640). Oxford: Oxford University Press.

Farrington, D. P. (2007b). Origins of violent behavior over the life span. In D. J. Flannery, A. J. Vaszonyi, & I. D. Waldman (Eds.), *The Cambridge handbook of violent behavior and aggression* (pp. 19–48). Cambridge: Cambridge University Press.

Farrington, D. P. (in press). Contextual influences on violence. In J. Dvoskin, J. L. Skeem, R. W. Novaco, & K. S. Douglas (Eds.), *Applying social science to reduce violent offending*. Oxford: Oxford University Press.

Farrington, D. P., Langan, P. A., & Tonry, M. (2004). *Cross-national studies in crime and justice.* Washington, DC: US Bureau of Justice Statistics (NCJ 200988).

Farrington, D. P., & Loeber, R. (1989). RIOC and Phi as measures of predictive efficiency and strength of association in 2 × 2 tables. *Journal of Quantitative Criminology, 5*, 201–213.

Farrington, D. P., & Loeber, R. (1999). Transatlantic replicability of risk factors in the development of delinquency. In P. Cohen, C. Slomkowksi, & L. N. Robins (Eds.), *Historical and geographical influences on psychopathology* (pp. 299–329). Mahwah, NJ: Lawrence Erlbaum.

Farrington, D. P., & Loeber, R. (2000a). Epidemiology of juvenile violence. *Child and Adolescent Psychiatric Clinics of North America, 9*, 733–748.

Farrington, D. P., & Loeber, R. (2000b). Some benefits of dichotomization in psychiatric and criminological research. *Criminal Behavior and Mental Health, 10*, 100–122.

Farrington, D. P., Loeber, R., Stallings, R., & Homish, D. L. (2008). Early risk factors for homicide offenders and victims. In M. J. Delisi & P. J. Conis (Eds.), *Violent offenders: Theory, research, public policy and practice* (pp. 79–96). Sudbury, MA: Jones and Bartlett.

Farrington, D. P., Loeber, R., & Stouthamer-Loeber, M. (2003). How can the relationship between race and violence be explained? In D. F. Hawkins (Ed.), *Violent crimes: Assessing race and ethnic differences* (pp. 213–237). Cambridge: Cambridge University Press.

Farrington, D. P., Loeber, R., Yin, Y., & Anderson, S. J. (2002). Are within-individual causes of delinquency the same as between-individual causes? *Criminal Behavior and Mental Health, 12*, 53–68.

Farrington, D. P., Ttofi, M. M., & Coid, J. W. (2009). Development of adolescence-limited, late-onset, and persistent offenders from age 8 to age 48. *Aggressive Behavior, 35*, 150–163.

Farrington, D. P., & Welsh, B. C. (2006). How important is "Regression to the Mean" in area-based crime prevention research? *Crime Prevention and Community Safety: An International Journal, 8*, 50–60.

Farrington, D. P., & Welsh, B. C. (2007). *Saving children from a life of crime: Early risk factors and effective interventions*. Oxford: Oxford University Press.

Farrington, D. P., & West, D. J. (1995). Effects of marriage, separation and children on offending by adult males. In J. Hagan (Ed.), *Current perspectives on aging and the life cycle* (Delinquency and disrepute in the life course, Vol. 4, pp. 249–281). Greenwich, CT: JAI.

Federal Bureau of Investigation. (2003). *Crime in the United States, 2001*. Washington, DC: FBI.

Federal Bureau of Investigation. (2008). *FBI, supplementary homicide reports, 1990–2008*. Washington, DC: FBI.

Fite, P. J., Wynn, P., & Pardini, D. A. (2009). Explaining discrepancies in arrest between black and white male juveniles. *Journal of Consulting and Clinical Psychology, 77*, 916–927.

Fleiss, J. L. (1981). *Statistical methods for rates and proportions* (2nd ed.). New York: Wiley.

Foreman, M. (2009). Preventable injuries burden State budgets. National conference of state legislators. *Legisbrief, 17*(3), 1–2.

Fox, J. A., & Zawitz, M. W. (2001). *Homicide trends in the United States*. Washington, DC: US Bureau of Justice Statistics.

Fox, J. A., & Zawitz, M. W. (2007). *Homicide trends in the U.S. Bureau of Justice Statistics*. Accessed from http://www.ojp.gov/homicide/race.htm.

Frick, P. J., O'Brien, B. S., Wootton, J. M., & McBurnett, K. (1994). Psychopathy and conduct problems in children. *Journal of Abnormal Psychology, 103*, 700–707.

Goodman, R. A., Mercy, J. A., Layde, P. M., & Thacker, S. B. (1988). Case-control studies: Design issues for criminological applications. *Journal of Quantitative Criminology, 4*, 71–84.

Hagelstam, C., & Häkkänen, H. (2006). Adolescent homicides in Finland: Offence and offender characteristics. *Forensic Science International, 164*, 110–115.

Hardwick, P. J., & Rowton-Lee, M. A. (1996). Adolescent homicide: Towards assessment of risk. *Journal of Adolescence, 19*, 263–276.

Harms, P. D., & Snyder, H. N. (2004, September). Trends in murder of juveniles: 1980–2000. *Juvenile Justice Bulletin.* Washington, DC: Office of Juvenile Justice and Delinquency Prevention.

Harpur, T. J., Hakstian, A., & Hare, R. D. (1988). Factor structure of the psychopathy checklist. *Journal of Consulting and Clinical Psychology, 56*, 741–747.

Harrendorf, S., Heiskanen, M., & Malby, S. (Eds.). (2010). *International statistics on crime and justice.* Helsinki: European Institute for Crime Prevention and Control; Vienna: United Nations Office on Drugs and Crime.

Hart, S. D., Cox, D. N., & Hare, R. D. (1995). *Manual for the psychopathy checklist: Screening version (PCL:SV).* Toronto, Canada: Multi-Health Systems.

Hawkins, J. D., & Catalano, R. F. (1992). *Communities that care.* San Francisco: Jossey-Bass.

Hawkins, J. D., Catalano, R. F., Kosterman, R., Abbott, R. D., & Hill, K. G. (1999). Preventing adolescent health-risk behaviors by strengthening protection during childhood. *Archives of Pediatrics & Adolescent Medicine, 153*, 226–234.

Hawkins, J. D., Kosterman, R., Catalano, R. F., Hill, K. G., & Abbott, R. D. (2005). Promoting positive adult functioning through social development intervention in childhood: Long-term effects from the Seattle Social Development Project. *Archives of Pediatrics & Adolescent Medicine, 159*, 25–31.

Hawkins, D. F., Laub, J. H., & Lauritsen, J. L. (1998). Race, ethnicity and serious juvenile offending. In R. Loeber & D. P. Farrington (Eds.), *Serious and violent juvenile offenders: Risk factors and successful interventions* (pp. 30–46). Thousand Oaks, CA: Sage.

Hawkins, J. D., Oesterle, S., Brown, E. C., Arthur, M. W., Abbott, R. D., Fagan, A. A., et al. (2009). Results of a type 2 translational research trial to prevent adolescent drug use and delinquency: A test of communities that care. *Archives of Pediatrics & Adolescent Medicine, 163*, 789–798.

Haynie, D. L., & Armstrong, D. P. (2006). Race- and gender-disaggregated homicide offending rates. *Homicide Studies, 10*, 3–32.

Heide, K. M. (1999). *Young killers: The challenge of juvenile homicide.* Thousand Oaks, CA: Sage.

Heide, K. M. (2003). Youth homicide: A review of the literature and a blueprint for action. *International Journal of Offender Therapy and Comparative Criminology, 47*, 6–36.

Heide, K. M. (2004). Juvenile homicide encapsulated. In A. R. Roberts (Ed.), *Juvenile justice sourcebook: Past, present, and future* (pp. 223–264). New York: Oxford University Press.

Highmark (2000). *Health care cost associated with violence in Pennsylvania 1994.* Camp Hill, PA: Human Services Research.

Holinger, P. C., Offer, D., Barter, J. T., & Bell, C. C. (1994). *Suicide and homicide among adolescents.* New York: Guildford.

Howell, J. C. (1998). Promising programs for youth gang violence prevention and intervention. In R. Loeber & D. P. Farrington (Eds.), *Serious and violent juvenile offenders: Risk factors and successful interventions* (pp. 284–312). Thousand Oaks, CA: Sage.

Howell, J. C. (2009). *Preventing and reducing juvenile delinquency.* Thousand Oaks, CA: Sage.

Hoyert, D. L., Arias, E., Smith, B. L., Murphy, S. L., & Kochanek, K. D. (2001). *Deaths: Final data for 1999.* Hyattsville, MD: National Center for Health Statistics.

Hrynkiw-Augimeri, L., Pepler, D., & Goldberg, K. (1993). An outreach program for children having police contact. *Canada's Mental Health, 41*, 7–12.

Huebner, B. M., Varano, S. P., & Bynum, T. S. (2007). Gangs, guns, and drugs: Recidivism among serious, young offenders. *Criminology & Public Policy, 6*, 187–221.

Huizinga, D., Thornberry, T. P., Knight, K. E., Lovegrove, P. J., Loeber, R., Hill, R. et al. (2006). *Disproportionate minority contact in the juvenile justice system: A study of differential minority arrest/referral to court in three cities.* Report to the Office of Juvenile

Justice and Delinquency Prevention. Accessed from http://www.ncjrs.gov/pdffiles1/ojjdp/grants/219743.pdf.

Ireland, J. L., Ireland, C. A., & Birch, P. (2009). *Violent and sexual offenders: Assessment, treatment and management*. Portland, OR: Willan.

Jessor, R., & Jessor, S. L. (1997). *Problem behavior and psychosocial development: A longitudinal study*. San Diego, CA: Academic.

Jolliffe, D., & Farrington, D. P. (2008). *The influence of mentoring on reoffending*. Stockholm, Sweden: National Council for Crime Prevention.

Kalson, S. (2010, January 20). Survey finds gun violence affects youth. *Pittsburgh Post Gazette*. Accessed from http://www.post-gazette.com/pg/10020/1029497-53.stm.

Kelly, K. D., & Totten, M. (2002). *When children kill*. Peterborough, Ontario: Broadview.

Koegl, C. J., Farrington, D. P., Augimeri, L. K., & Day, D. M. (2008). Evaluation of a targeted cognitive behavioral program for children with conduct problems-The SNAP under age 12 outreach project: Service intensity, age, and gender effects on short-and long-term outcomes. *Clinical Child Psychology and Psychiatry, 13*, 419–434.

Koolhof, R., Loeber, R., Wei, E. H., Pardini, D., & D'Escury, A. C. (2007). Inhibition deficits of serious delinquent boys of low intelligence. *Criminal Behaviour and Mental Health, 17*, 274–292.

Krug, E. G., Dahlberg, L. H., Mercy, J. A., Zwi, A. B., & Lozano, R. (2002). *World report on violence and health*. Geneva: World Health Organization.

Lauritsen, J. L., Laub, J. H., & Sampson, R. J. (1992). Conventional and delinquent activities: Implications for the prevention of violent victimization among adolescents. *Violence and Victims, 7*, 91–108.

Lauritsen, J. L., Sampson, R. J., & Laub, J. H. (1991). The link between offending and victimization among adolescents. *Criminology, 29*, 265–292.

Lewis, D. O., Lovely, R., Yeager, C., Ferguson, G., Friedman, M., Sloane, G., et al. (1988). Intrinsic and environmental characteristics of juvenile murderers. *Journal of the American Academy of Child and Adolescent Psychiatry, 27*, 582–587.

Lewis, D. O., Moy, E., Jackson, L. D., Aaronson, R., Restifo, N., Serra, S., et al. (1985). Biopsychosocial characteristics of children who later murder: A prospective study. *The American Journal of Psychiatry, 142*, 1161–1167.

Lipsey, M. W. (2003). Those confounded moderators in meta-analysis: Good, bad, and ugly. *The Annals of the American Academy of Political and Social Science, 587*, 69–81.

Lipsey, M. W., & Derzon, J. H. (1998). Predictors of violent or serious delinquency in adolescence and early adulthood: A synthesis of longitudinal research. In R. Loeber & D. P. Farrington (Eds.), *Serious and violent juvenile offenders: Risk factors and successful interventions* (pp. 86–105). Thousand Oaks, CA: Sage.

Lipsey, M. W., & Wilson, D. B. (1998). Effective intervention with serious juvenile offenders: A synthesis of research. In R. Loeber & D. P. Farrington (Eds.), *Serious and violent juvenile offenders: Risk factors and successful interventions* (pp. 313–345). Thousand Oaks, CA: Sage.

Lipsey, M. W., & Wilson, D. B. (2001). *Practical meta-analysis*. Thousand Oaks, CA: Sage.

Loeber, R., DeLamatre, M., Keenan, K., & Zhang, Q. (1998b). A prospective replication of developmental pathways in disruptive and delinquent behavior. In R. Cairns, L. Bergman, & J. Kagan (Eds.), *Methods and models for studying the individual* (pp. 185–215). Thousand Oaks, CA: Sage.

Loeber, R., DeLamatre, M., Tita, G., Cohen, J., Stouthamer-Loeber, M., & Farrington, D. P. (1999a). Gun injury and mortality: The delinquent backgrounds of juvenile victims. *Violence and Victims, 14*, 339–352.

Loeber, R., DeLamatre, M., Tita, G., Cohen, J., Stouthamer-Loeber, M., & Farrington, D. P. (1999b). Gun injury and mortality: The delinquent backgrounds of juvenile victims. *Violence and Victims, 14*, 339–352.

Loeber, R., & Dishion, T. (1983). Early predictors of male delinquency: A review. *Psychological Bulletin, 94*, 68–99.

Loeber, R., & Farrington, D. P. (Eds.). (1998). *Serious and violent juvenile offenders: Risk factors and successful interventions*. Thousand Oaks, CA: Sage.

Loeber, R., & Farrington, D. P. (2000). Young children who commit crime: Epidemiology, developmental origins, risk factors, early interventions, and policy implications. *Development and Psychopathology, 12*, 737–762.

Loeber, R., & Farrington, D. P. (Eds.). (2001). *Child delinquents: Development, intervention and service needs.* Thousand Oaks, CA: Sage.

Loeber, R., Farrington, D. P., Stouthamer-Loeber, M., Moffitt, T. E., Caspi, A., White, H. R., et al. (2003). The development of male offending: Key findings from 14 years of the Pittsburgh Youth Study. In T. P. Thornberry & M. D. Krohn (Eds.), *Taking stock of delinquency: An overview of findings from contemporary longitudinal studies* (pp. 93–136). New York: Kluwer/Plenum.

Loeber, R., Farrington, D. P., Stouthamer-Loeber, M., & van Kammen, W. B. (1998a). *Antisocial behavior and mental health problems: Explanatory factors in childhood and adolescence.* Mahwah, NJ: Lawrence Erlbaum.

Loeber, R., Farrington, D. P., Stouthamer-Loeber, M., & White, H. R. (2008). *Violence and serious theft: Development and prediction from childhood to adulthood.* New York: Routledge.

Loeber, R., Green, S. M., & Lahey, B. B. (1990). Mental health professionals' perception of the utility of children, mothers, and teachers as informants on childhood psychopathology. *Clinical Child and Adolescent Psychology, 19*, 136–143.

Loeber, R., & Hay, D. F. (1994). Developmental approaches to aggression and conduct problems. In M. Rutter & D. F. Hay (Eds.), *Development through life: A handbook for clinicians* (pp. 488–516). Oxford: Blackwell.

Loeber, R., & Hay, D. (1997). Key issues in the development of aggression and violence from childhood to early adulthood. *Annual Review of Psychology, 48*, 371–410.

Loeber, R., Keenan, K., & Zhang, Q. (1997). Boys' experimentation and persistence in developmental pathways toward serious delinquency. *Journal of Child and Family Studies, 6*, 321–357.

Loeber, R., Pardini, D., Homish, D. L., Wei, E. H., Crawford, A. M., Farrington, D. P., et al. (2005a). The prediction of violence and homicide in young men. *Journal of Consulting and Clinical Psychology, 73*, 1074–1088.

Loeber, R., Lacourse, E., & Homish, D. L. (2005b). Homicide, violence and developmental trajectories. In R. E. Tremblay, W. W. Hartup, & J. Archer (Eds.), *Developmental origins of aggression* (pp. 202–220). New York: Guilford.

Loeber, R., & Pardini, D. (2008). Neurobiology and the development of violence: Common assumptions and controversies. *Philosophical Transactions of the Royal Society B, 363*, 2492–2503.

Loeber, R., Pardini, D. A., Stouthamer-Loeber, M., & Raine, A. (2007). Do cognitive, physiological and psycho-social risk and promotive factors predict desistance from delinquency in males? *Development and Psychopathology, 19*, 867–887.

Loeber, R., & Stouthamer-Loeber, M. (1998). Development of juvenile aggression and violence: Some common misconceptions and controversies. *The American Psychologist, 53*, 242–259.

Loeber, R., Stouthamer-Loeber, M., Van Kammen, W. B., & Farrington, D. P. (1989). Development of a new measure of self-reported antisocial behavior for young children: Prevalence and reliability. In M. Klein (Ed.), *Cross-national research in self-reported crime and delinquency* (pp. 203–225). Dordrecht: Kluwer-Nijhoff.

Loeber, R., Wei, E., Stouthamer-Loeber, M., Huizinga, D., & Thornberry, T. P. (1999). Behavioral antecedents to serious and violent juvenile offending: Joint analyses from the Denver Youth Survey, Pittsburgh Youth Study, and the Rochester Youth Development Study. *Studies on Crime and Crime Prevention, 8*, 245–263.

Loeber, R., Wung, P., Keenan, K., Giroux, B., Stouthamer-Loeber, M., Van Kammen, W. B., et al. (1993). Developmental pathways in disruptive child behavior. *Development and Psychopathology, 5*, 101–132.

Lösel, F., & Beelmann, A. (2006). Child social skills training. In B. C. Welsh & D. P. Farrington (Eds.), *Preventing crime: What works for children, offenders, victims, and places* (pp. 33–54). Dordrecht: Springer.

Lynam, D. R., Caspi, A., Moffitt, T., Wikström, P.-O., Loeber, R., & Novak, S. (2000). The interaction between impulsivity and neighborhood context on offending: The effects of impulsivity are stronger in poorer neighborhoods. *Journal of Abnormal Psychology, 109*, 563–574.

MacDonald, J. M., & Gover, A. R. (2005). Concentrated disadvantage and youth-on-youth homicide. *Homicide Studies, 9*, 30–54.

Macintyre, S., & Homel, R. (1997). Danger on the dance floor: A study of interior design, crowding and aggression in nightclubs. In R. Homel (Ed.), *Policing for prevention: Reducing crime, public intoxication, and injury* (pp. 91–113). Monsey, NY: Criminal Justice Press.

Maguin, E., Zucker, R. A., & Fitzgerald, H. E. (1994). The path to alcohol problems through conduct problems: A family-based approach to very early intervention with risk. *Journal of Research on Adolescence, 4*, 249–269.

McCarty, C. A., Ebel, B. E., Garrison, M. M., DiGiuseppe, D. L., Christakis, D. A., & Rivara, F. P. (2004). Continuity of binge and harmful drinking from late adolescence to early adulthood. *Pediatrics, 114*, 714–719.

McGinnis, J. M., & Foege, W. H. (1993). Actual causes of death in the United States [see comments]. *Journal of the American Medical Association, 270*, 2207–2212.

Mercy, J. A., Rosenberg, M. L., Powell, K. E., Broome, C. V., & Roper, W. L. (1993). *Public health policy for preventing violence* (pp. 7–29). Winter: Health Affairs.

Miethe, T. D., & Regoeczi, W. C. (2004). *Rethinking homicide: Exploring the structure and process of underlying deadly situations*. Cambridge: Cambridge University Press.

Moffitt, T. E. (1993). Adolescence-limited and life-course-persistent antisocial behavior: A developmental taxonomy. *Psychological Review, 100*, 674–701.

Mokdad, A. H., Marks, J. S., Stroup, D. F., & Gerberding, J. L. (2004). Actual causes of death in the United States, 2000. *Journal of the American Medical Association, 291*, 1238–1245.

Nagin, D. S., Pogarsky, G., & Farrington, D. P. (1997). Adolescent mothers and the criminal behavior of their children. *Law and Society Review, 31*, 137–162.

Nieuwbeerta, P., McCall, P. L., Elffers, H., & Wittebrood, K. (2008). Neighborhood characteristics and individual homicide risk. *Homicide Studies, 12*, 90–116.

Olds, D., Henderson, C. P., Cole, R., Eckenrode, J., Kitzman, H., Luckey, D., et al. (1998). Long-term effects of nurse home visitation on children's criminal and antisocial behavior: 15-year follow-up of a randomized controlled trial. *Journal of the American Medical Association, 280*, 1238–1244.

Olds, D. L., Sadler, L., & Kitzman, H. (2007). Programs for parents of infants and toddlers: Recent evidence from randomized trials. *Journal of Child Psychology and Psychiatry, 48*, 355–391.

Pepler, D., Smith, P. K., & Rigby, K. (2004). Looking back and looking forward: Implications for making interventions work effectively. In P. K. Smith, D. Pepler, & K. Rigby (Eds.), *Bullying in schools: How successful can interventions be?* (pp. 307–324). Cambridge: Cambridge University Press.

Piquero, A. R., MacDonald, J., Dobrin, A., Daigle, L. E., & Cullen, F. T. (2005). Self-control, violent offending, and homicide victimization: Assessing the general theory of crime. *Journal of Quantitative Criminology, 21*, 55–71.

Poe-Yamagata, E., & Jones, M. A. (2000). *And justice for some: Differential treatment of minority youth in the justice system*. Oakland, CA: National Council on Crime and Delinquency.

Pope, C. E., & Snyder, H. N. (2003). *Race as a factor in juvenile arrests*. Washington, DC: Office of Juvenile Justice and Delinquency Prevention.

Raine, A. (1993). *The psychopathology of crime. Criminal behavior as a clinical disorder*. San Diego, CA: Academic.

Rivara, F. P., Ebel, B. E., Garrison, M. M., Christakis, D. A., Wiehe, S. E., & Levy, D. T. (2004). Prevention of smoking-related deaths in the United States. *American Journal of Preventive Medicine, 27*, 118–125.

Rivara, F. P., Shepherd, J. P., Farrington, D. P., Richmond, P. W., & Cannon, P. (1995). Victim as offender in youth violence. *Annals of Emergency Medicine, 26*, 609–614.

Roberts, A. R., Zgoba, K. M., & Shahidullah, S. M. (2007). Recidivism among four types of homicide offenders: An exploratory analysis of 336 homicide offenders in New Jersey. *Aggression and Violent Behavior, 12*, 493–507.

Rosenfeld, R. (2009). Crime is the problem: Homicide, acquisitive crime, and economic conditions. *Journal of Quantitative Criminology, 25*, 287–306.

Roth, R. (2009). *American homicide*. Cambridge, MA: Harvard University Press.

Sampson, R. J., & Lauritsen, J. L. (1990). Deviant lifestyles, proximity to crime, and the offender-victim link in personal violence. *Journal of Research in Crime and Delinquency, 27*, 110–139.

Schaeffer, C. M., & Borduin, C. M. (2005). Long-term follow-up to a randomized clinical trial of multisystemic therapy with serious and violent juvenile offenders. *Journal of Consulting and Clinical Psychology, 73*, 445–453.

Schweinhart, L. J., Montie, J., Zongping, X., Barnett, W. S., Belfield, C. R., & Nares, M. (2005). *Lifetime effects: The high/scope Perry preschool study through age 40.* Ypsilanti, MI: High/Scope Press.

Siegel, J. E., Weinstein, M. C., Russell, L. B., & Gold, M. R. (1996). Recommendations for reporting cost-effectiveness analyses. *Journal of the American Medical Association, 276*, 1339–1341.

Snyder, H. N., & Sickmund, M. (1995). *Juvenile offenders and victims: A focus on violence.* Pittsburgh: National Center for Juvenile Justice.

Snyder, H. N., & Sickmund, M. (1999). *Juvenile offenders and victims: 1999 national report.* Washington, DC: Office of Juvenile Justice and Delinquency Prevention.

Snyder, H. N., & Sickmund, M. (2006). *Juvenile offenders and victims: 2006 national report.* Washington, DC: Office of Juvenile Justice and Delinquency Prevention.

Spelman, W. (2000). The limited importance of prison expansion. In A. Blumstein & J. Wallman (Eds.), *The crime drop in America* (pp. 97–129). Cambridge: Cambridge University Press.

Stephan, J. J. (2004). *State prison expenditures, 2001.* Washington, DC: US Department of Justice (NCJ 202949).

Stouthamer-Loeber, M., Creemers, J., Loeber, R., Homish, D. L., & Wei, E. (2001a). *Juvenile justice and mental health interventions for juveniles who eventually commit homicide.* Paper presented at the meeting of the American Society of Criminology, Atlanta, GA.

Stouthamer-Loeber, M., Loeber, R., Homish, D. L., & Wei, E. (2001b). Maltreatment of boys and the development of disruptive and delinquent behavior. *Development and Psychopathology, 13*, 941–955.

Stouthamer-Loeber, M., Loeber, R., & Thomas, C. (1992). Caretakers seeking help for boys with disruptive and delinquent child behavior. *Comprehensive Mental Health Care, 2*, 159–178.

Stouthamer-Loeber, M., Loeber, R., Wei, E., Farrington, D. P., & Wikstrom, P.-O. (2002). Risk and promotive effects in the explanation of persistent serious delinquency in boys. *Journal of Consulting and Clinical Psychology, 70*, 111–123.

Stouthamer-Loeber, M., Wei, E., Homish, D. L., & Loeber, R. (2002). Which family and demographic factors are related to both child maltreatment and persistent serious juvenile delinquency? *Children Services: Social Policy, Research, and Practice, 5*, 261–272.

Strom, K. J., & MacDonald, J. M. (2007). The influence of social and economic disadvantage on racial patterns in youth homicide over time. *Homicide Studies, 11*, 50–69.

Teplin, L. A., McClelland, G. M., Abram, K. M., & Mileusnic, D. (2005). Early violent death among delinquent youth: A prospective longitudinal study. *Pediatrics, 114*, 1586–1593.

Theobald, D., & Farrington, D. P. (2009). Effects of getting married on offending: Results from a prospective longitudinal survey of males. *European Journal of Criminology, 6*, 496–516.

Theobald, D., & Farrington, D. P. (2010). Should policy implications be drawn from research on the effects of getting married on offending? *European Journal of Criminology, 7*, 239–247.

Thornberry, T., & Krohn, M. (2003). *Taking stock of delinquency.* New York: Kluwer.

Tolan, P. H., Gorman-Smith, D., & Loeber, R. (2000). Developmental timing of onsets of disruptive behaviors and later delinquency of inner-city youth. *Journal of Child and Family Studies, 9*, 203–230.

Tremblay, R. E., Nagin, D. S., Seguin, J. R., Zoccolillo, M., Zelazo, P. D., Boivin, M., et al. (2004). Physical aggression during early childhood: Trajectories and predictors. *Pediatrics, 114*, 43–50.

Tremblay, R. E., Pagani-Kurtz, L., Masse, L. C., Vitaro, F., & Pihl, P. O. (1995). A bimodal preventive intervention for disruptive kindergarten boys: Its impact through mid-adolescence. *Journal of Consulting and Clinical Psychology, 63*, 560–568.

Tuma, F., Loeber, R., & Lochman, J. E. (2006). Introduction to special section on the National Institute of Mental Health State of the Science Report on violence prevention. *Journal of Abnormal Child Psychology, 34*, 451–456.

U.S. Department of Health and Human Services. (2000). *Healthy People 2010*. Washington, DC: Government Printing Office.

van der Laan, A., Blom, M., & Kleemans, E. R. (2009). Exploring long-term and short-term risk factors for serious delinquency. *European Journal of Criminology, 6*, 419–438.

van Soest, D., Park, H. S., Johnson, T. K., & McPhail, B. (2003). Different paths to death row: A comparison of men who committed heinous and less heinous crimes. *Violence and Victims, 18*, 15–33.

Webster, C. D., & Hucker, S. H. (2007). *Violence risk. Assessment and management*. Chichester: Wiley.

Webster-Stratton, C. (1998). Preventing conduct problems in Head Start children: Strengthening parenting competencies. *Journal of Consulting and Clinical Psychology, 66*, 715–730.

Webster-Stratton, C., Mihalic, S., Fagan, A., Arnold, D., Taylor, T. K., & Tingley, C. (2001). *Blueprints for violence prevention, book eleven: The incredible years-parent, teacher, and child training series*. Boulder, CO: Center for the Study of Prevention of Violence.

Weinrott, M. (1975). *Manual for retrieval of juvenile court data*. Eugene, OR: Evaluation Research Group. Unpublished manuscript.

Weinstein, M. C., Siegel, J. E., Gold, M. R., Kamlet, M. S., & Russell, L. B. (1996). Recommendations of the panel on cost-effectiveness in health and medicine. *Journal of the American Medical Association, 276*, 1253–1258.

Welsh, B. C., & Farrington, D. P. (2010). Effective programs to prevent delinquency. In J. R. Adler & J. M. Gray (Eds.), *Forensic psychology: Concepts, debates and practice* (2nd ed., pp. 378–403). Cullompton, Devan: Willan.

White, H. R., Jackson, K., & Loeber, R. (2009). Developmental sequences and comorbidity of substance use and violence. In M. Krohn, A. Lizotte, & G. P. Hall (Eds.), *Handbook of deviance and crime* (pp. 434–468). *New York: Springer Publications*.

White, H. R., Loeber, R., Stouthamer-Loeber, M., & Farrington, D. P. (1999). Developmental associations between substance use and violence. *Development and Psychopathology, 11*, 785–803.

Wideman, J. E. (2005). *Brothers and keepers*. Boston: Houghton Mifflin.

Wikström, P.-O., & Treiber, K. H. (2009). Violence as situational action. *The International Journal of Conflict and Violence, 3*, 75–96.

Wikström, P.-O., & Loeber, R. (2000). Do disadvantaged neighborhoods cause well-adjusted children to become adolescent delinquents? A study of male juvenile serious offending, individual risk and protective factors, and neighborhood context. *Criminology, 38*, 1109–1142.

Wilson, M. N., Hurtt, C. L., Shaw, D. S., Dishion, T. J., & Gardner, F. (2009). Analysis and influence of demographic and risk factors on difficult child behaviors. *Prevention Science, 10*, 353–365.

Wolfgang, M. (1958). *Patterns of criminal homicide*. Philadelphia, PA: University of Pennsylvania Press.

Zagar, R. J., Busch, K. G., Grove, W. M., & Hughes, J. R. (2009). Summary of studies of abused infants and children later homicidal, and homicidal, assaulting later homicidal, and sexual homicidal youth and adults. *Psychological Reports, 104*, 17–45.

Index

A
ACME data. *See* Allegheny County Medical
    Examiner's data
Age-crime curve
  arrest, violence, 138
  disruptive/delinquent behavior, 138
  Federal Bureau of Investigation, 140
  intervention
    at-risk status, 151
    delinquent acts, frequency of, 142
    high-risk participants, 144
    homicide offenders and victims, 141
    incarceration, 142
    justice system, 147
    limitations, 151–152
    offense rate/frequency, 149
    robbery/assault, 144
    self-reported serious delinquents, 147
    serious violence and theft, 142
    simulation research, 141
    timings, 150
    young age, 146
  juvenile court data, 140
  police arrest, 140
  screening device, 137
  simulation representation, 139
Allegheny County
  African American residents, 42
  gang-related homicide, 45
  geographic mapping and cluster analysis,
    44
  guns, 45
  homicide rates, 42
  offenders' motivation, 45
  Pittsburgh neighborhoods, 43
  police data, 45
  shooting clusters, 44

Allegheny County Medical Examiner's
    (ACME) data, 39
Antisocial potential (AP), 171

C
Convicted homicide offenders
  African American boys, 75
  behavioral predictors
    logistic regression analysis, 63
    risk factors, 64
  childhood risk factors
    attitude, 60
    behavior, 60
    child-rearing, 59
    dichotomization, 60
    dose–response relationship, 58
    neighborhood, 59–60
    parental, 59
    peer delinquency, 60
    school, 60
    socioeconomic status, 59
  explanatory predictors, 61–62
  homicide arrestees, 66–67
  integrated homicide risk score, 74–75
  logistic regression analysis, 73
  overprediction, 72–73
  previous criminal history, 57
  prior criminal offenses, 76
  psychopathy, 76
  racial differences, 63
  risk scores, 77
  screening risk score, 65–66
  young age
    arrests, 71
    arrests and convictions, 68
    convictions, 70

Convicted homicide offenders (*cont.*)
    criminal risk score, 71
    drug and alcohol abuse, 68
    illegal economy, 69
    logistic regression analyses, 72
    property arrests, 70
    self-reported delinquency, 69
Convicted homicide offenders and controls
    demographic factors, 116–117
    drug usage, 118
    gangs, 117–118
    measures, 116
    methods, 115–116
    psychopathy, 118–119
    self-reported delinquency, 117
    situational factors
        co-offenders, 120
        offense setting, 119
        reasons, offense, 119
        timings, 120
        weapons, 120

F

Federal Bureau of Investigation (FBI), 140

G

Geographic information system (GIS), 44

H

Homicide and shooting victims
    aggression, reciprocal process of, 96
    behavioral predictors
        homicide offenders, 101
        risk score, 101
        screening risk score, 101–102
        serious delinquency, 100
    childhood predictors
        African American males, 96
        antisocial behavior, 97
        prediction analyses, 96
    criminal predictors
        convicted homicide offenders, 105
        convictions, 103
        logistic regression analyses, 104
        number of arrests, 105, 106
        self-reports, 103
    explanatory predictors
        callous-unemotional behavior, 98
        homicide offenders, 99
        race, 99–100

    risk score, 98–99
    illegal activities, 96
    integrated prediction
        logistic regression analysis, 106, 107
        risk score, 106–107
    longitudinal studies, 95
    shooting victims
        antisocial behavior, 108
        attitudinal factors, 109
        comparison, 111
        race, 108
        risk score, 110–111

I

Integrated cognitive antisocial potential
        (ICAP) theory, 171–172
Interventions and policy
    causal process, 167–168
    comparison, 163, 168–170
    convicted homicide offenders
        and victims, 153
    criminal predictors, 168
    developmental and life-course theories
        antisocial methods, 172
        attachment and socialization
            process, 173
        disadvantaged neighborhoods, 175
        ICAP theory, 171
        illicit property transactions, 175
        long-term AP, 171
        neighborhood influences, 174
        personal justice, 176
        property crime, 174
        short-term AP, 173
        situational factors, 171
    homicide arrestees, 159
    homicide offenders
        African Americans, 155
        behavioral predictors, 156–157
        callous-unemotional behavior, 158
        criminal predictors, 157
        criminal record, 155
        dose–response relationship, 158
        explanatory predictors, 156
        logistic regression analysis, 159
        marijuana, 156
        prediction analyses, 158
        psychopathy, 158
        step-wise prediction, 159
        street homicides, 155
    homicide victims, 161–162
    incarceration and waiver, 179–180

interpersonal conflict, 170
limitations, 154
national and local initiatives, 184–185
Pittsburgh, 183–184
preventive interventions
    age–crime curve, arrests, 182
    disruptive/delinquent behavior, 182
    high-risk populations, 183
    homicide offending and violence, 180
    mental health services, 180
    multisystemic therapy, 181
    Nurse Home Visitation Program, 181
    Perry Preschool Program, 181
race, 176–177
screening and risk/needs assessment,
    178–179
shared predictors, 163–164
shooting victims, 162–163
socioeconomic factors, 169
univariate predictors, 163
violent offenders, 160–161

M
Multisystemic therapy (MST), 129

N
National homicide rate
aggressive behavior, 123
childhood and adolescence
    decision analysis, 131
    early childhood education, 129
    longitudinal follow-up data, 128
    multisystemic treatment, 129
    nurse home visiting, 128
    school-based intervention programs,
        129
    therapeutic foster care, 129
    violence prevention intervention, 128
childhood education program, 132
data sources
    incarceration costs, 127
    index crime, 125
    juvenile justice data, 128
    prior violent history, 127
    violence prevention decision model,
        126–127
decision analysis, 131–132
early home visitation programs, 132
homicide deaths, 125
incarceration, 123
multisystemic therapy, 132

parameter estimation, 124
PYS, 124–125
randomized trials, 124
years of potential life lost (YPLL), 125
youth violence prevention, 123
National Rifle Organization (NRA), 2

P
Pittsburgh youth study (PYS)
cohorts characteristics, 21
convicted homicide offenders
    drug dealing, 53
    gang-related homicide, 52–53
    guns, 51
    homogeneous, 52
    manslaughter, 51
    multiple-perpetrator homicides, 51
    retaliation, 53
    robbery, 52
design, 19–20
extent of follow-ups, 21
homicide offenders and victims
    African American males, 50
    ages, 48
    aggravated assaults, 40
    alleged offenses, 49
    arrest history, 54
    Caucasians, 50
    conviction rate, 48
    criminal records, 47
    nonoffending, 54
    Pennsylvania and Allegheny
        County, 39
    prior arrest/criminal record, 41
    relationships, 41
    revenge, 54–55
    robbery, 54
    USA, 38
    victimization, 47
    violence trends, 39–40
    years of, 49
measurements and constructs
    birth factors, 32
    child attitudes/cognition, 26–27
    child behavior factors, 25–26
    child psychiatric diagnoses, 27
    child's history of offending, 28–32
    demographic factors, 35–36
    family factors, 32–34
    peer factors, 34
    school factors, 35
screening, 20

Pittsburgh youth study (PYS) (*cont.*)
  violence, developmental pathways
    causation, 23–24
    homicide, 21
    overt pathway, 22
    physical aggression, 22
    problem behaviors, 23
    race and violence, 24
    secular changes, 23
    selection process, 22
    serious theft, 23
Psychopathy checklist-screening version
  (PCL-SV), 118

V
Violent boys
  African American race, 91
  antisocial behaviors, 93
  arrested/convicted homicide offenders
    risk score, 91–92
  child behavior problems/ truancy, 82
  convicted homicide offenders
    explanatory factors, childhood, 89
    homicide risk score, 88
    independent predictors, 87
    predictors, 83–84
  disruptive behavior disorder, 82
  dose–response relationship, 80, 85
  earlier analyses, 79
  gang reduction programs, 94
  long-term risk factors, 93
  multiple regression analyses, 85
  predictive efficiency, 80
  preventive interventions, 93

  racial/ethnic differences, 82
  risk factors, 82
  self- reported violent/nonviolent
    offending, 92
  stepwise prediction, 79
  true prediction estimation,
    89–90
  violence risk score, 85
Vulnerable individuals
  case-control publications, 3
  criminal justice system, 2
  evil act, 1
  gun violence, 2
  health and justice records, 2
  homicide offenders and violent offenders
    African American youth, 3
    arrest, 9–10
    court records, 5
    hand guns, 4
    illegal economy, 5
    mental illness, 5
    Pittsburgh community, 4
    prediction, 7
    prospective longitudinal surveys, 6
    retrospective reports, 6
    risk factors, 7
    street crime-driven homicides, 5
    theories, 14–15
    types, 8–9
    United States, 3
  homicide victims, 10–11
  incarceration *vs.* prevention, 15–17
  PYS, 5
  screening, 12–13
  shooting victims, 11–12

CPSIA information can be obtained at www.ICGtesting.com
Printed in the USA
LVOW030545220911

247352LV00007B/46/P